What Are People Sayir

This book Greg has taken time to write not only gives you an idea of the exceptional time he has given to serve our great Nation from the Coast Guard Academy to upholding Law and Order on an unprecedented scale, he shares unique experiences that don't have a name or stamp as they are so rare. When a man like Greg Shaffer, with a background as unique as his takes the time to pen a book, for your safety, its more than just another "author." The words so effortlessly read, come from one of the most secretive and highly trained people in the world, you will help yourself and family by the purchase of this exceptional read.

Consider this: There are 330-million people in the United States. Less the one-million of those are in law enforcement, less than fifteen thousand are in the FBI working as special agents. Now consider the FBI's Elite Hostage Rescue Team (HRT), where Greg was a member for a great deal of time. That unit has had less than 400 members who've ever donned the name and the title "HRT Operator." Again, when someone works for a specialized unit that has a total club number of less than 400, that's "TOTAL" and is rich in its intriguing history, from training and missions most will never fully realize, it's the "go to" for a lesson and in how to help yourself and family. Offering more than just daily safety tips, there's an exceptional personal travel security chapter that few could reduce to such rational print... This offered by "one humbled contributor."

Chris Grollnek MS/AJS, Retired
Active Shooter Prevention Expert
Author | Media Contributor | Public Speaker

In a day of greatly increased violence and terrorism, *Stay Safe* immediately puts worthwhile tools directly into the hands of everyday citizens. It will educate and equip not only those in the security field but also the parent taking their child to school. Further, *Stay Safe* will familiarize the reader with certain principles that will help guide their actions in the midst of chaos.

Brig Barker, CEO/Red Rock Global Security Group
FBI Supervisory Special Agent (Retired)

Do not buy one copy of this book. Buy a copy for everyone you care about. *Stay Safe* is the definitive work on personal, family, and business security. I learn something every time I browse through it. I will be buying copies for my family and clients.

Danny O. Coulson
Deputy Assistant Director FBI, Retired
First Team Commander of the FBI's HRT
Author | Media Contributor | Public Speaker

Recommendations

Greg and I met in 2012. During our first lunch, we talked intensively about fear. More exactly, Greg spoke and I listened. It was clear to me, this man feared little. Greg's background ensured that he could keep his cool in the most difficult situations. That's the kind of person I want to learn from.

William Benko, Hungarian American Entrepreneur

In HR we deal with all walks of life, and as you know, there are some dangerous characters in the work force. Greg's expertise, instruction, and knowledge have enabled me to identify possible threats in the workplace, as well as being prepared for whatever may come our way at the office or at home.

Lance Turner, HR Executive

I have personally witnessed Greg's superb performance and I know of his high standing reputation in the FBI community. He is head and shoulders above a pack of very talented and devoted agents. Greg has distinguished himself at every opportunity throughout his law enforcement career. His most recent endeavor at Shaffer Security Group is another example of his superior performance. Greg is the complete package, a proven law enforcement expert, with broad meaningful experience and an uncanny ability to bring others willingly up to his level. When operational success is on the line, Greg Shaffer is the person you want out front.

Jack Santucci, Captain USCG, Retired
Gulfstream G550/G650 Captain, Safety Officer
Certified Aviation Manager—
National Business Aircraft Association

I first worked with Greg during Super Bowl XLV and recently took his Active Shooter and Personal Safety Awareness course. Greg is able to modify his approach in order to reach an audience of all backgrounds, from the security expert to the grandmother next door who volunteers at a local community center. Whether you are traveling overseas to a new location or seeking to improve situational awareness in your daily environment, the skill set Greg teaches is invaluable and can be well adapted to any situation.

Lisa Chambers
Former CIA
Southeast Asia Subject Matter Expert

STAY SAFE

STAY SAFE

security secrets for
today's dangerous world

GREG SHAFFER

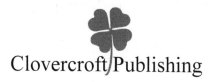

Clovercroft Publishing

About the Title

The title Stay Safe came as a result of my thirty-one years in law enforcement. When police officers set forth on their assignments each day, it is common practice to reinforce the fact that their jobs are inherently dangerous. Therefore, often the last thing said to their fellow officers as they set out, is the reminder to "Stay Safe."

Published by Clovercroft Publishing, Franklin, Tennessee in association with Results Faster Publishing, Flower Mound, Texas.

Copy Editor: Christy Callahan

Cover Design by Andrea McNeeley

Interior Design by Adept Content Solutions

Printed in the United States of America

978-1-948484-57-2

Dedicated to the men and women
of law enforcement.

Thank you for putting others before self
and for your dedication, commitment,
and honor to serve and protect.

Stay Safe!

CONTENTS

PREFACE

People often ask me, "Why did you join the FBI?" Honestly? I think it's in my DNA. I have always believed there are some professions that choose you; you don't choose them. I don't believe you just decide one day to *become* a teacher or a doctor or a cop. You teach children, treat the sick, or serve the citizens and arrest the bad guys because it is *who you are*. I knew from a very early age that I wanted to serve in the military and be an FBI special agent. It was in my nature, a part of my soul. It was almost as if I didn't have a choice. Being an FBI Agent was my calling. It was just who and what I am.

So, who am I? I am a product of great parents! My dad was a great father, and my mother was a charming and beautiful woman—they were married for 51 years. I grew up in a *Leave It to Beaver* or *Father Knows Best* type of household. We went to church every Sunday, opened every door for my mother, prayed before each meal, stood at attention for the National Anthem, and said thank you to police officers and firefighters. My favorite uncle was one of my dad's younger brothers, Uncle Dick. Uncle Dick served in Vietnam, and my brothers and I would try to get him to tell stories about his service. He only told us the funny stories and never divulged the horrors of war that he witnessed, which tragically haunted him until his early death. I do remember him giving me his boonie hat one summer when I was about ten years old. I must have worn that thing every day for years. When I wasn't wearing it, it was hanging on my bed post. Although my Dad never served in the military—he married my mom at the age of nineteen and had the first of five sons at age twenty, so Vietnam was not an option for him—he did instill a sense of patriotism and love of one's country that eventually propelled me to my future in the FBI.

My father worked for IBM, which meant we moved every three years. Most people believe IBM stands for International Business Machine, when in fact those working for the company know it stands for "I've Been Moved"! Because we relocated as often as we did, my brothers and I developed a close relationship and learned to trust each other as we attended new schools and tried to make new friends. My older brother and I are only thirteen months apart and are quite close. We grew up playing whatever sport was in season—fall football; winter basketball; spring baseball. We loved playing cops and robbers, Americans vs. Germans or cowboys and Indians, and we would ask for a new BB gun every Christmas.

One day in April 1980, my older brother and dad came running up to the baseball field in Wanaque, New Jersey, where I was pitching a game for the Lakeland Regional High School "Lancers". They both had these huge grins on their faces, and when the inning ended, they came to the dugout and handed me my letter of acceptance to the US Coast Guard Academy. It was one of the happiest days of my life!

Military academies, whether it's West Point, Annapolis, Air Force Academy, or Kings Point, are not programmed to be enjoyed. For the entire first year (known as Swab Year or Plebe Year) I was running to every class and every meal. I was required to "make chins" at all times (pulling my chin into my chest); I had to memorize three meals in advance and recite the menus upon request. I needed to know what movies were playing at the local theater, memorize the specifications of the M-16 rifle and Colt .45 sidearm, and recite the details of every class of Coast Guard Cutters and aircraft in operations. It was at the USCG Academy where my love of country blossomed. I loved every minute of it!

After four years at CGA (Coast Guard Academy) I not only received a bachelor of science degree, but I had also been schooled in leadership skills, basic marksmanship, shipboard firefighting, survival skills, celestial navigation, coastal navigation, and other "tradecraft skills" that would serve me later in the FBI.

From 1986–1988, I was selected to command the US Coast Guard Cutter *Point Steele* (WPB-82359), an eighty-two-foot patrol boat homeported in Fort Myers Beach, Florida. Commanding the *Point Steele* was one of the highest honors I have received in my blessed life. With a crew of ten, we spent our days and nights hunting for drug smugglers and conducting search and rescue missions in the Gulf of Mexico. As captain, or "Skipper" as the crew called me, I could not have been more proud of the Gulf Coast Men of Steele (our ship's motto). These dedicated young Coast Guardsmen were truly some of America's finest. The *Point Steele* conducted hundreds of search and rescue missions during my two-year command, and we saved hundreds of lives and millions in property. But the most fun we had was doing offshore drug interdiction operations. The *Point Steele* had multiple drug seizures, the largest of which was over forty tons of marijuana. Most of our drug seizures was a direct result of DEA intelligence. Having to testify after these seizures put me in direct contact with the DEA special agents who worked the "sources" that provided the intelligence on the drug-laden vessels. With that information, the *Point Steele* would intercept, board, and seize the vessel and arrest its crew. Again, I loved every minute of it!

It was during this time the DEA started to recruit me, telling me stories about what it was like being a "Fed," conducting undercover operations, arresting bad-guys and thriving on life-and-death situations. I was hooked!

I started to do some research on various federal law enforcement agencies—USSS, DEA, BATF, CIA, CBP, and the FBI. During this time, my younger brother was hired by the USSS (US Secret Service). After many interviews, polygraphs, written tests, panel interviews, physical exams, physical fitness evaluations, and a yearlong background check, I chose the FBI—or rather they chose me!

It was 1995 when I joined the Bu (special agent slang for the FBI). The five months of New Agent Training in Quantico, Virginia, were awesome—who doesn't like to shoot guns and drive fast cars? All the while I was learning Title 18 of the United States Code (the main criminal code of the federal government). It was during this time I met my first HRT operator. I had never heard of the HRT (Hostage Rescue Team) prior to arriving in Quantico. Once I started my training to be a FBI special agent, I was able to learn a little more about those quiet professionals who stayed to themselves on their fenced-in and gated compound, at the edge of the FBI Academy. I learned that the dark helicopters, which often flew very low in the dark of night, were filled with HRT operators conducting training. Whenever an FBI Academy Instructor (Senior FBI special agents) talked of the HRT, it was almost in reverence and in a hushed tone. I wasn't totally sure who these men were in their black flight suits walking around the Academy with a certain swagger and a whole lot of confidence—but I knew I wanted to be one!

My first interaction with an HRT operator was in Pickel Meadows, California, at the US Marine Corps Mountain

Warfare Training Center (MWTC) in 1996. The MWTC was located twenty-one miles northwest of Bridgeport, California, at an elevation of 6,800 feet, in the Toiyabe National Forest. It was also the site for the San Francisco FBI Special Weapons and Tactics (SWAT) team's mountain climbing and winter survival training. I was selected (after a very difficult tryout) to be a member of the FBI San Francisco SWAT Team very shortly after arriving in the San Francisco Division. The FBI was just starting a new program called the Enhanced SWAT Team program. Seven FBI Divisions were selected to be a part of this enhancement, which allowed these seven SWAT teams to man, equip, and train up to forty SWAT operators. San Francisco was selected as part of this program when I arrived as a newly badged FBI special agent; they were also doubling the number of SWAT team operators. The Bureau's rule that a special agent needed to have two years of field experience before you can try out for SWAT was not enforced if you had prior law enforcement or military experience. Due to my time in the USCG, I was able to try out for the SWAT team after only two months as an FBI special agent.

One of the benefits of being on an Enhanced SWAT Team was it received "Advanced SWAT Training" from the finest operators in the world—the HRT. While in Pickel Meadows the HRT sent some of their helicopters (MD 540 Little Birds) and a few Operators and pilots to assist in the training of the San Francisco SWAT team. These HRT operators were hardened professionals, yet generous with their knowledge. At the conclusion of the training, I was even more convinced I wanted to be a part of this extraordinary group of professionals.

The FBI Hostage Rescue Team (HRT) is a true "Tier One" National Security Council asset. The HRT is on par with both the US Navy's Special Warfare Development Group, better known as SEAL Team 6, and with the US Army Special

Operations Command, Combat Activities Group (CAG), better known as DELTA Force. I would never compare myself or my experiences with my many friends and colleagues on both SEAL Team 6 and CAG (Delta Force)—they are true American heroes and badasses; however, I do know the HRT routinely operates side by side with these men and have done so since the HRT's inception. The very first HRT operators, known as Generation One, were sent down to Fort Bragg and were trained by the then very secret, unacknowledged Delta Force. To this day the HRT enjoys a very close relationship with that amazing group of warriors. The HRT has operated in Iraq, Afghanistan, Yemen, Somalia, Libya, and other nondisclosed locations. The HRT is the only *nonmilitary* Tier One tactical unit in the US arsenal. Because it is not a military unit, it can operate domestically, on US soil, without violating the Posse Comitatus Act (18 USC 1385), which prevents federal military personnel from enforcing domestic policies within the United States.

The HRT was established as a direct result of the 1972 Munich Olympics Hostage Crisis. During the 1972 Summer Olympic Games, eleven Israeli Olympic team members were taken hostage and eventually killed, along with a German police officer, by the Palestinian terrorist group Black September. All the athelete-hostages were killed during a botched rescue attempt conducted by the German police at the Munich airport.

By 1972 the United States had already been awarded the 1980 Lake Placid Winter Olympic Games and the 1984 Los Angeles Summer Olympic Games. President Nixon convened his National Security Council and asked them what the US response would be should a similar terrorist attack occur in either Lake Placid or Los Angeles. His question was answered with silence. The United States did not have a national asset that was capable of this type of high-speed, hostage rescue. In 1972, SEAL Team 6 did not exist and DELTA Force was so secretive the US government refused to acknowledge its existence. Besides, as mentioned earlier, the Posse Comitatus Act prevents the US military from enforcing laws on US soil. President Nixon realized the country needed a highly trained, well-equipped unit that was able to conduct hostage rescue operations domestically. He instructed the FBI to develop such a team—hence, the genesis of the Hostage Rescue Team.

I actually tried out for the HRT on two separate occasions. My first selection was in 1997. We started with over forty selectees, and had only ten standing at the end of the grueling selection process. Of the ten remaining, the Team chose six—I was not one of the six chosen. Not to be dissuaded, in the spring of 1999 I returned to Quantico for my second attempt to make the Team. I'm not going to lie; knowing what to expect—the mind games and the distances of some of the runs—certainly made my second selection easier. However, I also knew what a "kick in the nuts" I was about to put my body through, and that made the second attempt more difficult.

In the summer of 1999 I relocated from San Francisco, California, to Quantico, Virginia, to begin what was arguably the best six years of my life—as an HRT operator with the call sign "Alpha Niner Six."

From 1999 through 2005, I was a part of something bigger than I could have ever imagined. I say this without hesitation; the men of the FBI's Hostage Rescue Team are the bravest, most professional, intelligent, and selfless men this great country has to offer. There have been fewer than four hundred men to ever call themselves HRT—the pride I have in serving with these men, these heroes, is immeasurable.

The training at HRT is second to none. No expense is spared in providing the operators with the finest equipment, most advanced gear, and the highest caliber of training the world has to offer. There were many days during New Operator Training

School, known as NOTS, where we would shoot over one thousand rounds a day. Imagine the blisters on my thumbs as I loaded thousands upon thousands of rounds of ammunition into various magazines for the many different weapons, months on end. By the end of NOTS I was a true surgical shooter, and an expert in firearms and close quarter battle (CQB). I received advanced training in trauma medicine, satellite communications, explosives, driving, diving, skydiving, tracking, and surviving in all environments. It is rumored over a million dollars goes into the training for each operator during NOTS.

My experiences on HRT are mostly classified. Those that are not included the hunt and apprehension of the DC Snipers, Lee Boyd Malvo and John Mohammed, the hunt for the USS Cole bombers, Usama bin Laden, Saddam Hussein, and a host of other bad actors and world terrorists. I've conducted tactical operations in Iraq, Yemen, the Philippines, Saudi Arabia, Indonesia, Kenya, Tanzania, Greece, and other parts of the globe. I've trained and operated with the finest Counter Terrorism Teams in the world, and worked side by side with US Navy SEALS, the US Army's Special Operations Command, the US Secret Service, US Marshals, DEA, CIA, DHS, Border Patrol, and the brave men and women of local and state law enforcement.

After six years of world travel and excitement, I decided to leave HRT and head a few miles north to McLean, Virginia, site of the newly established National Counter Terrorism Center—the NCTC. Established in 2004, the NCTC was a direct result of the lack of communication in the US Intelligence Community (IC), specifically between the FBI and CIA, during the planning of the 9/11 attacks. The 9/11 Commission, which analyzed the failings of our intelligence and investigated the terrorist attack of September 11, 2001, concluded "none of the measures adopted by the US government before 9/11 disturbed or even delayed the progress of al Qaeda in planning their attack."

As a result of 9/11, many things changed, particularly within the FBI. The Bureau's entire paradigm shifted from that of a law enforcement agency, which conducts investigations after an incident, to a domestic intelligence agency that collects data and intelligence and prevents incidents from happening. Laws were changed, presidential (executive) orders were signed, and the agencies that make up the Intelligence Community were placed in one building. Lack of communication would never again allow us to miss an attack plan against our nation. The NCTC houses multiple agencies, including the CIA, FBI, NSA, DHS, DEA, BATF, USMS, USAF, USN, USA, USMC, USCG, USSS, Department of Energy, Department of State, Defense Intelligence Agency, National Reconnaissance Office, and the NYPD.

When I took the promotion to the NCTC, I knew I was walking into the belly of the beast. Working long hours with some of the greatest minds in the IC was both rewarding and eye-opening. Seeing how Counter Terrorism (CT) Operations run at eye level and on the battlefield is what I did for six years on the Team. Seeing how CT Operations run at the 35,000 foot level was something totally different. It was fascinating to see the intelligence come in from hundreds of different, unrelated sources and tie into one evil plot to kill Americans. Then, we'd watch the process as our IC partners collected additional intelligence using FISA warrants, undercover agents, then developed link charts that would connect hundreds of people in dozens of countries all involved in a single evil plot to kill "infidels." It was truly amazing to be a part of the genesis of the NCTC and witness the evolution of what is now the most effective Intelligence Community in the world.

After about two years of NCTC work, I got burned out. Long hours spilling over data and intelligence reports, as well as talking to undercover agents, sources, and foreign law enforcement partners caused serious brain melt! I needed to find a new position to maintain my sanity. My pay-pack assignment for volunteering to go into the belly of the beast was I could pick and choose any office in the FBI. I chose Dallas, Texas.

I was assigned as a supervisor on the North Texas Joint Terrorism Task Force (NTJTTF). Here, I managed terrorism investigations in North Texas as well as managed the special event security and counter terrorism planning. Large-scale public events have always been a target for terrorists. When it comes to large scale, no one does it bigger or better than Texas. Part of my responsibilities was to design, plan, implement, and manage the security for large-scale, public events held in North Texas. During my tenure on the NTJTTF (2007–2011) I planned and supervised the security for the 2011 NFL Super Bowl, 2011 NBA World Championship Series, 2010 NBA All Star Game, 2010 MLB World Series, the annual Cotton Bowl, Armed Forces Bowl, Texas Rangers MLB Opening Day, multiple NASCAR events at Texas Motor Speedway, multiple PGA events, airshows, and a host of other events deemed to be potential targets of terrorism. Of course, this was a team effort, and I had a lot of help from some outstanding FBI Agents, as well as top-notch, professional, and dedicated local and state law enforcement. The 2011 Super Bowl security plan involved over eighty different law enforcement agencies! Truly an honor to work with each and every one! They say you are only as good as the people around you. Well, I was surrounded by the most professional, intelligent and bravest men and women in law enforcement.

After four years in Dallas, with my children in college or out of the house, my wife and I decided we needed some more adventure. I requested to be the FBI Director's designate as the Bureau's first Legal Attaché in Budapest, Hungary. Over ninety US Embassies worldwide now have an FBI Legal Attaché office, known as LEGATS. In June of 2011, we started our Hungarian adventure; and what an adventure it was. We were living in one of the most beautiful cities of the world with incredible history and even more charming people. As the Legal Attaché, I was the senior FBI agent-in-country. I was working in our United States Embassy, a senior staff member of our US ambassador, and assisting the Hungarian National Police. Living in Budapest afforded my wife and me the opportunity to travel Europe and many other parts of the world where we enjoyed the history, the various cultures, and the many fine wines. When we left Budapest after our three-year assignment, we both left a large part of our hearts in Hungary. We still remain good friends with several Hungarian police families and Hungarian citizens. Not a day goes by that I don't think of Budapest, its stunning beauty, and its captivating people.

With only one more year until I was eligible to retire, we decided to return to Dallas. This time, I was not interested in supervising special agents or managing security for Super Bowls. I vowed to leave the FBI in the same manner in which I started—kicking in doors and arresting bad guys! I asked to be assigned to the Violent Crimes Task Force (VCTF). My last year in the FBI was as much fun as my first year. My squad served warrants and made arrests on a daily basis. We hunted and arrested Dallas' most violent criminals. A special thanks to my squad supervisor and my ASAC (Assistant Special Agent-in-Charge) who let me do what I do best—catch the bad guys! And to the men and women on the VCTF Squad, thanks for having my back! Stay safe.

In June of 2015, after thirty-one years and two months of government service, I decided to leave Uncle Sam and start my own security consulting firm. With a lot of love and support from my incredible wife, Dotty, and the help, guidance, and instruction from great men like Larry Shaffer (older brother),

Danny Coulson, Brian Harpole, and Chris Grollnek, Shaffer Security Group (SSG) was launched.

At Shaffer Security Group (SSG), our philosophy is simple: SSG was created for the protection and security of our clients' assets and interests. Our goal is to train and educate employees, staff members, and teach the general public that **"survival is not a skill set; it is a mindset!"**

My hope in writing *Stay Safe* is to help you protect everything you hold dear and to teach you how to respond swiftly and effectively regardless of the crisis situation.

Evil exists ... stay safe!

INTRODUCTION

Evil exists.

On June 12, 2016, Omar Mateen, a twenty-nine-year-old security guard, walked into Pulse Nightclub in Orlando, Florida, and killed forty-nine people. The death toll makes this attack one of the worst terrorist events on US soil since 9/11.

The official After-Action Report of this horrific shooting revealed that thirteen people died while hiding together in the club's two restrooms. Nine waited in one restroom; four waited in another.

I was not present during this horrendous murder spree, but I can imagine that the level of fear and terror in that nightclub must have been paralyzing for some. I can't help but wonder: What would have happened if those young men and women, huddled in the restroom, had banded together, developed a plan, and pounced on the shooter as soon as he entered the bathroom? Instead, the thirteen victims most likely were frozen in fear, unable to act, and waited for their turn to die. What prevented those young men and women from fighting back?

Had I been at the Pulse Nightclub on that tragic night, I do know Mr. Mateen would not have found me helplessly hiding in the bathroom stall. No, Mr. Mateen would have entered that restroom, and we would have attacked him as if our lives depended on it.

In a world of ever-increasing mass shootings and terrorist attacks, we must be prepared to respond quickly, wisely, and instinctively. My hope in writing this book is that if, God forbid, you ever find yourself in a similar situation, you will be equipped with the knowledge, mental preparedness, and assuredness to formulate a plan and act.

As a former FBI agent with over thirty years of experience in counterterrorism, counternarcotics, hostage rescue, and security planning, I've learned, lived, and taught the tactics and techniques that, if used correctly, could save your life in a crisis situation.

Stay Safe will teach you to be more situationally aware, more in tune with your gut instinct, and more prepared to fight or flee to save your life and those around you in crisis situations. Whether you are at the theater or your child's school play; in a taxi or in your car; at work or at home; online or on a plane, this book will teach you how to be prepared both mentally and physically and how to respond in a crisis.

Stay Safe is not about teaching you hand-to-hand combat, Jiu Jitsu, or ground-fighting skills. Those skills take years of practice and thousands of repetitions before they're effective. It won't make you a quasi-FBI agent or a tactical gun fighter. Rather, this book will teach you how to recognize indicators prior to an attack and what actions to take to keep you safer in today's more dangerous world. We will cover topics such as **personal security** and **situational awareness, improvised weapons, travel security, active shooter response, special event security,** and much more.

When I am hired as a security consultant, risk manager, tactical firearms instructor, or travel safety advisor to C-level executives, the most difficult aspect of my job is getting good people to understand that evil people exist.

My intention in writing *Stay Safe*, is to teach you tactics, techniques, and procedures taught to Tier One operators, CIA operatives, FBI special agents, undercover agents, and others, which will allow you to be situationally aware and able to **effectively respond** to any crisis or violent incidents you or your family might face.

And, most of all, to *Stay Safe*!

Part 1
"STAY SAFE" PRINCIPLES

Chapter 1
THE SURVIVAL MINDSET

W hen evil visits and danger lurks in the shadows, **survival is not a skill set; it is a mindset.**

In the Pulse Nightclub massacre, what was it that prevented those young adults from banding together and fighting to the death? The situation was truly a "fight or die" situation once the shooter entered the restroom. We will never know the answer, but we do know most people's gut response is to not fight back. For the average person, the *Survival Mind*-set, even in a "kill or be killed" situation, does not instinctually kick in.

We saw the same response in some of the victims in the 2007 Virginia Tech shooting where thirty-two innocent people were slaughtered. One survivor of the Virginia Tech massacre said, "I laid on the floor and waited for my turn to die." The Virginia Tech shooter is known to have reloaded his weapon several times in some of the classrooms. Why didn't those uninjured students attack the shooter while he was reloading? Why didn't anyone fight back? Once the shooter entered the classroom, why didn't they get up from their desks and run out the door? What was their mindset that prevented the survival instinct from taking over and fighting with all their might, or running as fast as they could?

3

We need to reevaluate what we are teaching our children. As a society, have we become negligent in our child rearing, raising a generation who allow themselves to be slaughtered? For us to teach our children that evil does not exist, or that fighting is unjust, is doing them a disservice. In fact, it is getting our children killed!

By refusing to believe that evil may visit our lives and by insulating our children from the horrors of the world, or by rationalizing that "it will never happen to me," is getting us killed. We are not mentally preparing ourselves should terror strike, which makes us easy fodder for the real evil that does exist. Omar Mateen was evil. There are more like him.

It's time we start developing a new attitude for ourselves and to instill in our children. An attitude that clearly states, "I will fight you with all that I have to protect my life or the lives of those I love." That is a *Survival Mindset*.

The will to survive beats the skill to survive.

You need certain skills to survive, and this book will teach you many of those skills. However, all the survival skills in the world will not help you survive if you are not mentally prepared to use those skills.

Survival is a mindset.

More than equipment, training, or skill, survival for a Tier One operator is first and foremost a mindset. All Naval Special Warfare Operators (SEALS), US Army Special Operations Command Operators (DELTA Force), or a good SWAT cop have one thing in common: their mental resiliency, or "mental toughness." Every one of these warriors truly believes there is no one, absolutely no one, who can kill them. A warrior believes no one will best him or her. It is not bravado or conceit or pride; it's a mindset that makes them believe they are invincible. There is nothing these warriors will not do to succeed or to win. As a former member of the FBI's elite Hostage Rescue Team (HRT), I know how hard these men train. They train mercilessly. Warriors are always learning and trying to improve their skill set.

> Warriors aren't born and they aren't made; they create
> themselves through trial and error. And by their
> ability to conquer their own frailties and faults.
> — Philip J. Messina

If it's true that warriors create themselves, what is preventing you from becoming a warrior? The first step in that creation is developing a mental attitude that you will not be a victim; you will not be defeated; you will stand up and fight in the face of evil and violence. Start developing that *Survival Mindset* as you continue to read this book.

Expert marksman Clint Smith, founder of the famous firearms range, Thunder Ranch, and former US Marine, is renowned for his humorous, yet thoughtful, quotes on fighting. One of my favorites is: "If you find yourself in a fair gunfight, you're not cheating hard enough." Now, that is a mindset!

While I am not advocating everyone learn how to use a firearm to defend themselves, this quote applies regardless of what kind of fight you are in.

"Cheating," you ask?

Yes, cheating is certainly allowed if you're fighting for your life!

Mr. Smith continues, "There are no rules in a fight for life or death! You do everything in your power to win that fight." If you lose, it will be the last poor decision you will ever make. To lose is to die! On the flip side, Mr. Smith also states, "There are only two rules in a fight; always cheat and always win."

So, this brings me to my next point: Are you prepared to cheat and to win? Are you mentally able to do whatever it takes to survive? Have you rehearsed it in your mind or "role played" how you would survive? Have you consciously said aloud, "In the event I am being violently assaulted, I will fight back and do whatever it takes to survive"? Do you have the mindset to attack and possibly kill another human being if your life or the lives of those you love depended on it? If the day ever comes when you are faced with fighting for your life, I want you to have the confidence to know, no matter the situation, you have the knowledge and mindset to respond appropriately in any crisis situation.

There is a quote I use at the end of every class I teach: *"If violence is the last resort, you better be good at it!"*

Think about it. Violence can only be stopped by more violence. You cannot talk your way out of an active shooter event where the sociopath's intent is to kill as many innocent people as he can. The only way to stop the killing is to kill the offender.

Here is the situation: you have a gun pointed at your face, the offender is a stone cold killer, and your life comes down to this moment and one final question—do you "hope" or do you "act"? Do you hope he doesn't shoot you in the face, or do you take an action to prevent him from shooting you in the face?

There is a highly acclaimed book written by Lieutenant Colonel Dave Grossman, titled *On Combat: The Psychology and Physiology of Deadly Conflict in War and in Peace* (Grossman 2004).

This book is a virtual Bible for every law enforcement officer, special warfare operator, and self-made warrior. It is a must read for anyone serious about surviving violent encounters. In his book Lt. Col. Grossman uniquely and succinctly describes the psychological and physiological responses to high-threat, high-stress life-or-death situations. I highly recommend this book to anyone who truly wants to understand what it is like to be in combat without actually having to be there.

In his chapter "On Sheep, Wolves, and Sheepdogs," Lt. Col. Grossman writes there are three kinds of people in the world—Sheep, Wolves, and Sheepdogs. He states that over 90 percent of the world can be classified as Sheep—and there is nothing wrong with that. These people are law-abiding citizens; they love peace and quiet, they do the right thing, go about their lives, and are unlikely to strike back should violence strike.

Another segment of society can be classified as Wolves. Wolves are vicious creatures. They will attack a person just because they wanted their wallet or decided to rape someone. They are evil, often sociopaths. They often kill for the thrill of it. Remember, **evil exists!**

Fortunately, there is a third kind of person in the world—Sheepdogs. Much like the Sheep, Sheepdogs prefer peace; however, they are aware that there is evil in the world. Sheepdogs know the Wolves prowl about looking for Sheep to devour. Sheepdogs do not crave violence and wish the world were free of murders, rapes, and assaults. But they know evil exists and they train to protect the Sheep when the Wolf attacks. The Sheepdog hones his skills in order to take his or her stand against those who perpetrate violence.

The irony is, Sheep generally do not like the Sheepdog. He looks a lot like the Wolf. Both the Sheepdog and the Wolf are canines. They both have fangs; they both have the capacity for violence; and they are both capable of killing the Sheep. The difference is the Sheepdog must not, cannot, and will not, ever harm the Sheep. Any Sheepdog who intentionally harms a lamb will be put to death.

As Grossman writes, "The Sheep would much rather have the Sheepdog cash in his fangs, spray paint himself white, and go, 'Baa.' That is, until the Wolf shows up. Then, the entire flock desperately tries to hide behind the one lone Sheepdog." Still, the Sheepdog disturbs the Sheep. He is a constant reminder that there are Wolves lurking among us.

Understand that there is nothing morally superior about being a Sheepdog; it's just what you choose to be. Also understand that a Sheepdog is a funny creature. He is always sniffing around out on the perimeter, checking the breeze, barking at things that go bump in the night, and yearning for a righteous fight.

Here is how the Sheep and the Sheepdog think differently. The sheep pretend the Wolf will never come, but the Sheepdog lives for that day. After the attacks on September 11, 2001, most of the Sheep, that is, most citizens in America said, "Thank God I wasn't on one of those planes." The Sheepdogs (Warriors) said, "Dear God, I wish I had been on one of those planes. Maybe I could have made a difference." When you are truly transformed into a warrior and have truly invested yourself into "warrior-hood," you want to be there—in the fight, defeating evil. You want to be able to make a difference.

Being a Sheepdog does have one real advantage. He is able to survive and thrive in an environment that can destroy 98 percent of the population. Had one Sheepdog been trapped in the restroom with eight other patrons at the Pulse Nightclub, Mr. Mateen's murderous rampage may have ended the moment he entered the restroom.

Here is the point I like to emphasize, especially when speaking to the thousands of police officers and civilians as I do each year: In nature, real sheep are born as sheep. Sheepdogs are born as sheepdogs, and wolves are born as wolves. They didn't have a choice in what they were. But you, as a human being on top of the food chain, can be whatever you want to be. It is a conscious, moral decision. Be a Sheepdog!

Grossman tells us if you want to be a Sheep, then you can be a Sheep, and that is okay; but you must understand the price you might pay. If the Wolf comes, you and your loved ones may suffer if there is not a Sheepdog in your midst to protect you. If you want to be a Wolf, you can be one, but the Sheepdogs are going to hunt you down and you will never have rest, safety, trust, or love. But if you want to be a Sheepdog and walk the warrior's path, then you must make a conscious and moral decision every day to dedicate, equip, and prepare yourself for that toxic, corrosive moment when the Wolf comes knocking at the door.

Many off-duty police officers carry their weapons when they go to church on Sunday morning. I do as well. My weapon is concealed, and no one would ever know I was armed, unless the Wolf appeared. Should the Wolf enter my place of worship and attempt to bring his brand of violence, I would end his life without remorse. You may never know if there is such an individual in your church, school, office, playground, or shopping mall, until the Wolf appears to slaughter you and the Sheepdog springs into action.

As you read stories of tragedies, watch the latest action movie, or see news programs on the most recent active shooter event (ASE), you may often find yourself asking, "Why did they react that way?" or, "Why didn't anyone do something?" If you think these questions, then you are on your way to becoming the "Sheepdog." You will be the warrior who organizes those around you during a crisis and develops a solution to end it. I urge you to keep reading, there is so much more you are going to learn.

Survival Mindset is having the confidence to know, no matter the situation, that you possess the knowledge and mindset to respond appropriately in any crisis situations.

How to Develop the Survival Mindset

I am often asked, "How do I develop the Survival Mindset?" The answer is in the question; that is, you *develop* it. No expert in his or her field has ever mastered their craft by hoping and wishing. It was through hard work, dedication, commitment and training they were able to become *experts in their field*. It is no different in training yourself to develop your survival mindset.

The first step is to read and study examples of human survival in what would normally be considered un-survivable situations. One recommendation is to read the incredible story of survival of Louis Zamperini, as detailed in Laura Hillenbrand's book *Unbroken*. Research stories where the human mind and body survived insurmountable odds. Gain "domain knowledge" on the subject of survival mindset.

Actionable things you can do to develop a survival mindset include the following:

Arousal Control

You must take responsibility and teach yourself how to control your state of arousal. It is the ability to ramp up or tone down your level of arousal to suit the circumstances. This is critical for your initializing and sustaining the right action that best suits the crisis you are facing. Can you control your panic response? It is necessary to survive most critical incidents, and you can train yourself to control your arousal response.

Attention Control

This is the ability to broaden and narrow your attention beam to enable you to fully account for and respond to all the variables in a critical incident. **Tunnel Vision** and **Weapon Focus** are two examples of how our normal physiological response to stress can inhibit or enhance our chances of survival. Train yourself to look and see. I have witnessed on many occasions at the gun range, my students looking at a target, but not seeing the weapon in the hand. See and understand what you're looking at. Collecting information is useless if you do not know how to process it. The ability to process this information is what enhances your survival mindset.

Imagery

Visualization is a skill to use in critical situations to help you maintain that survival mindset. Any master in the realm of sports, law enforcement, or the military knows the importance of imagery and having finely honed skills to mentally rehearse various situations in their heads. You must imagine your course of action prior to taking action. Visualization can be used to quickly process a situation and develop the right strategy to resolve the crisis.

"The body can't go where the mind has never been" is a frequently used saying in the security world. You must mentally rehearse the actions you want to take in a critical incident to ensure your survival. Your chances of making the right decision without playing it out in your mind beforehand are minimal. Always ask yourself, "What would I do if ... (insert critical incident here)."

Self-Talk

Maintain a positive attitude and survival mindset by talking to yourself. Use personal mantras that help maintain positive thinking patterns under pressure. Even something as simple as "keep moving" can help lift your spirits and keep you focused on surviving in the face of danger. I can't count the number of times I have talked my way through difficult situations.

Goal Setting

We all know the importance of setting goals in life. They help us to achieve things we desire and give us a plan that we can follow to achieve those goals. In a crisis situation, goal setting is even more important. Short-term goals to survive the next five minutes keep us focused in controlling our fears. Long-term goals may be to survive until tomorrow. In a survival situation, create easily achievable goals that keep your mindset in check.

To Move Is to Live—To Freeze Is to Die

In any armed confrontation or an active shooter event, the best piece of advice I can give you is, *Move! Walk away! Run! Get off the X* (the spot or location where the violence is occurring). Your first response should always be to remove yourself from the situation!

I know how hard it can be to just walk away. Trust me; my pride has gotten the better of me on more than one occasion. Having the good sense to walk away from a potential confrontation shows you are in control and have the sense to make good choices.

My wife and I were out on date night one evening in downtown Baltimore, near the Inner Harbor. The Inner Harbor is a beautiful area of Baltimore, next to the historic brickstone baseball park where the Orioles play. It's on the water with a fantastic maritime museum, and a variety of great eating establishments.

On this evening, my wife and I were walking, hand in hand, along the waterfront and found ourselves only a block or two away from the main tourist area. Realizing we had wandered a bit too far off the tourist path, my senses quickly heightened. My "Situational Awareness" (discussed in the next chapter) was immediately in tune with my surroundings. As we turned around and started walking back toward the "safer" areas, we saw two men come around the corner about a hundred feet away, stare us straight in the eye, and walk directly toward us. I felt my wife squeeze my hand a little tighter before I released it and quietly told her to stay close to me. The distance between the two strangers and us was closing. I led my wife off the sidewalk and started to cross the street to gain separation between the two men and us. As we started to alter our direction, I could tell the two men were about to follow us into the street. When they were about twenty feet away, I looked them in the eye, raised my hand over my shoulder in a wave, put a big smile on my face, and said, "Hey guys! How you doing? Great to see you again."

Both men instantly and involuntarily flinched, mumbled back at me, "Hey dude," and altered their movement back onto the sidewalk as my wife and I continued to cross the street. My wife looked at me and asked, "You know those guys?" I smiled and said, "Never seen them before in my life." So exactly what happened to make those men flinch, alter their direction and, in my opinion, decide not to attempt to victimize us? Answer: moving into the street, making good eye contact, asking a direct question, and resetting their decision-making process is key.

The point is, I didn't let my ego get in the way. Was I armed at the time? Absolutely. Could I have escalated the situation and made things a lot more dangerous by verbally challenging them—or pull back my jacket to expose my weapon and FBI badge affixed to my waist? You better believe it. What I chose to do was move off the X and defuse the situation with a little human psychology. Was I confident in my ability to address this threat had it escalated? Certainly. But by verbally addressing the threat, making eye contact, asking a direct question, and implying that I knew them, I was able to de-escalate a potentially dangerous situation, all the while moving off the X.

There is an important point to remember in any physical confrontation: You have a 50 percent chance of getting seriously injured in any kind of fight. You never know who your adversary may be or know his mindset, his background, his training, or his propensity to use extreme violence. Always walk away from a fight! Only engage when you have absolutely no other means of de-escalation and no escape. And when you are forced to engage, use extreme violence!

When Violence Is the Answer

In *When Violence is the Answer—Learning How to Do What it Takes When Your Life is at Stake* (2017), author Tim Larkin states that violence is rarely the answer, but when it is, it's the *only* answer. It is essential to understand this statement when developing your "Survival Mindset." Violence is almost never the answer, but when it is, it is the only answer! When your life is threatened with extreme, asocial violence, you must throw out the "rule book" and do whatever has to be done to survive. Often this means using the "tool" of violence. You can only implement this tool with the right mindset.

Extreme raw bloody violence can and does permeate all demographic lines, be it race, gender, religion, nationality or socioeconomic status. None of us are immune to violence once an offender has identified us as his target. I understand and fully appreciate that a bigger, stronger, and more muscular person, who fully intends to do serious bodily harm, can trigger a base fear in any of us. It's natural to try to push those fears to the back of our minds, especially when we know we don't possess the knowledge or the skills to properly defend ourselves. Instead we justify our fears by telling ourselves, "It will never happen to me."

I am here to tell you that that approach is wrong! The solution to this base fear is not denial or rationalization; it is knowledge and preparedness that creates confidence. This confidence will then produce the right "mindset."

In his book, Larkin teaches that an effective strike against your adversary is one that causes a debilitating injury that takes your opponent's most valuable weapon, his brain, out of the equation and destroys any advantage that strength, size, or musculature may give him. He details the principles on how to do this throughout his book. Larkin clearly explains how to develop these principles and thereby defeat a man who is stronger, bigger, and faster. I highly encourage you to read it. I have encouraged my wife and daughters to read it knowing it could save their lives in the event they are ever caught in a violent situation. When it comes to trauma to the human body, all men are created equal—we all have the same vulnerable areas such as the throat, eyes, knees, groin, elbows, and seventy other targeted sites.

As a society, we usually associate violence with criminals. We tell ourselves that since violence is used by criminals, it must be criminal itself. Therefore, violence is evil, violence is bad. Not necessarily! Violence is a tool—nothing more, nothing less. Whether it's a criminal doing unspeakable violent acts who uses a gun or knife, or the victim who uses that same weapon to defend himself, it's still the same gun or knife. The weapon works in the hands of the victim equally well as it does in the hands of the violent offender. The weapon has no intent or decision-making abilities. It does not pick sides; it does whatever the person holding it wants it to do. It can be used for good or for evil, to kill or to save a life.

When your life is at stake at the hands of a violent offender and you have no means of escape, you need to come to the complete understanding that violence is the only tool that will save your life. There is no sanitized version of violence where it is not so bloody, or doesn't hurt as much. A screwdriver used in self-defense driven into the eye of a would-be rapist looks just like a screwdriver driven into the eye of an innocent murder victim. Although violence is often ugly, it is just a tool.

Of all the animals, man is the only one that is cruel. He's the only one to inflict pain for the pleasure of doing it.
—Mark Twain.

Random violence happens! We don't have to embrace it, condone it, like it, or even understand it; but we must accept that it is a part of today's world. People hurt other people, sometimes fatally. Remember, evil exists.

You cannot negotiate with true violence. You cannot talk your way out of the hands of a serial killer. Violent offenders, like Omar Mateen or Ted Bundy, do not care about your social status—they just want to maim, kill, and destroy you, and those with you. Understanding that reality, and training your mind to deal with these unlikely encounters, will give you the confidence you need to quickly and calmly identify the situation and render your assailant incapacitated, unconscious, or dead. In a violent encounter, your only course of action to save your life is to do what your assailant is trying to do to you, but do it more quickly, effectively, efficiently, and do it first—to use the very same tool of violence.

You do not have to wait for the attacker to make the first move. You should not be constrained by any social rules of aggression, because your asocial violent offender is unconstrained by any sense of right and wrong. If violence becomes inevitable and inescapable, or if you are trapped with nowhere to safely retreat, do not hesitate—attack! Attack without remorse, without pity, and without a second thought. Make it count and don't stop until the threat is neutralized, or you can escape.

Those who survive violent encounters do so because they have the mindset and the intent to do real harm to another human when real harm is what's required. Larkin's book, *When Violence Is the Answer*, will teach you exactly how to do this.

Four Percent "Hit Rate"

You're going to hear me say this a lot: To move is to live; to freeze is to die. As you read about the many crisis situations people have faced throughout this book, you will see that it is those who move are those who survive. Here is why I am a firm believer that movement saves lives. I am an expert shooter. I am very proficient with all types of firearms, particularly with a handgun and a carbine. But I prefer handgun shooting. To this day I still go to the gun range at least once a week to shoot a couple hundred rounds with my Glock handguns. I still compete in shooting matches and love my time shooting steel in combat training courses. The finest shooters in the country have trained me, including Jerry Barnhart, Ken Hackathorn, Jerry Miculek, and Scott Warren (the Principal Firearms Instructor at HRT during my time on the Team). During NOTS (New Operator Training School), when I was learning to become an HRT operator, there were many days where we would shoot over one thousand rounds of ammunition a day! Why am I telling you all of this? Because I know how to shoot, and I also know how hard it is to hit a moving target with a handgun. The hit rate for an assailant with a weapon hitting a moving target is 4 percent! Yes, 4 percent, and the kill rate is less than 1 percent. So, even with a gun stuck in your face, your best chance of survival is to get off the X: Move! Walk Away! Run! The chances of you being critically injured are LESS THAN 1 PERCENT.

By getting off the X, you are also disrupting the assailant's decision-making process, which significantly increases your chances of survival in a crisis situation. We will discuss in detail in the next chapter how this works.

The Gift of Fear

Gut Instinct. Women's Intuition. Your Inner Voice. Whatever you call it, we all have it and if you listen to it, it could save your life!

In his award-winning and best-selling book, *The Gift of Fear: Survival Signals That Protect Us from Violence* (1997), author Gavin DeBecker interviews survivors of very violent crimes. During his research, he found almost all of those victims who survived violent encounters had a "bad feeling" or a "gut instinct" that warned them something horrible was about to happen. Had these survivors listened to their inner voice, or their "gift of fear," they may have been able to avoid what was probably the worst moment of their lives.

Although everyone has this advanced warning system, most people dismiss the feeling or rationalize their fears away. People will tell themselves they're being paranoid; or they don't want to embarrass themselves or their would-be attacker. Most people tell themselves, "It won't happen to me" or, "I'm just being silly." The key is this: the gift of fear is based on external stimuli that you may not be able to articulate or identify or describe. Remember, your gut instinct reflects your best interest—it will not deceive you.

Pre-Incident Indicators

Everyone has the innate ability to pick up on the signals and signs that someone will become violent. A person may explode and become violent, but often the fuse is lit long before the actual violence takes place. These pre-incident indicators, identified by DeBecker, are essential in maintaining your Situational Awareness to prevent you from possible violent encounters:

- **Forced teaming:** A person implies that they have something in common with their chosen victim, acting as if they have a shared predicament when that isn't really true. Speaking in "we" terms is a mark of this, such as, "We don't need to stay here. Let's go somewhere else." Or, "We should go now. This party is lame!"
- **Charm and niceness:** A stranger being overly polite and friendly to a chosen victim in order to manipulate them by disarming their distrust.
- **Too many details:** If a person is lying they will add excessive details to make themselves sound more credible to their chosen victim when in fact they're adding details because they know their story is not true.
- **Typecasting:** A slight insult is used to get the victim to prove it isn't true, or to engage in conversation to counteract the insult. For example: "You're too beautiful to go out with a guy like me." The tendency is for the chosen victim to want to prove the insult untrue.
- **Loan sharking:** Giving unsolicited help to the chosen victim, anticipating they'll feel obliged to extend some reciprocal openness in return.
- **The unsolicited promise:** A promise to do (or not to do) something when no such promise is asked for; this usually means that such a promise will be broken. For

example, an unsolicited "I promise I'll leave you alone after this" usually means the chosen victim will not be left alone. Similarly, an unsolicited "I promise I won't hurt you" usually means the person intends to hurt their chosen victim.

- **Discounting the word "no."** Refusing to accept rejection; not recognizing the word "no."

The Gift of Fear is full of case histories of stalkers who turned violent or of co-workers who went on a shooting spree. DeBecker convincingly highlights how these tragedies could have been averted had the signs, which were clearly there, been picked up and acted upon.

There's a fantastic comparison in the beginning of *The Gift of Fear* that really brought things into perspective for me. DeBecker relates the intuition of humans to animals. Our intuitive abilities are far superior to that of animals because we add to our experiences each day. The difference between man and animal is, we have "judgment" and animals do not.

Judgment skews our perception and intuition when it comes to fear. It causes us to disregard our gut instinct unless we can explain it *logically*. No animal in the wild would suddenly be overcome with fear and then spend the next ten minutes thinking, "It's probably nothing." In contrast to every creature in nature, humans choose to explore—and even ignore—signs of danger. I call this judgment influence "rationalization." Rationalizing irrational behavior is how we as humans cope with fear, unwanted change, or undesirable circumstances. We are wired to fear change and try to normalize the situation to fit our own desires.

My favorite example of rationalization is when a television reporter interviews witnesses of an active shooter event. "What did you think when you first heard the shots ring out?" the reporter almost always asks. The response of most witnesses, "I thought it was fireworks." Really? If I were the news reporter, my follow-up question would be, "How many times have fireworks been lit off in your work place?" In the active shooter instance, the witness decides it can't be gunfire because it would be an irrational act to fire any weapon in an office building. As human beings we rationalize the "fear of gunfire" in our workplace as being anything *except* gunfire! In many active shooter situations, those killed have often left an area of safety to go and investigate the sound of gunfire. The victims hear the gunfire, but mentally cannot accept the fact they're hearing gun shots in their work-place – they rationalize that it cannot be gunfire, and are killed as a result.

Don't be caught rationalizing things that are too uncomfort-able for you to admit to seeing or hearing. Unless it's the Fourth of July, if you think you hear fireworks, think gunfire instead. Then, take appropriate action. Being knowledgeable and under-standing the need to listen to your "inner voice" is critical to avoid crisis situations or high-threat confrontations.

Never distrust your gut instinct. You are not paranoid. Your body can pick up on bad vibrations and indicators you may tend to dismiss or ignore. If something deep inside of you says something is not right about a person or situation ...TRUST IT.

Chapter 2
SITUATIONAL AWARENESS

S erial killer Ted Bundy once stated that he could spot a victim by the way she walked down the street, by the tilt of her head or the manner in which she carried herself.

The FBI's Behavioral Analysis Unit (BAU) is a group of the world's foremost experts in profiling serial killers and understanding what makes them do the horrific things they do. There are numerous studies that have looked at how and why criminals select their victims. As a result, there is a pretty accurate picture of what criminals look for in choosing their next victim. What are the behaviors that tell a serial killer someone is vulnerable to victimization? Some of the most recent research on the subject confirms a very startling hypothesis.

In criminal behavioral studies, serial killers and violent offenders have been asked how they choose their victims. A lot of the typical answers are related to matters of natural selection, such as comparative physical size or stature, perceived situational awareness (which we will discuss further in this chapter), whether or not they are alone, and their gender.

A recent study in the *Journal of Interpersonal Violence* shows the criteria used in selecting a victim are much less encompassing (Book, Costello, and Camilleri, 2013). This new study shows that body language and walking pattern are key factors in victim selection.

The basic idea of the study was to show inmates videos of selected individuals walking down a sidewalk and rate their perceived vulnerability. The selected individuals also provided testimony stating whether or nor they had ever been victims of a violent crime. The result was the inmates gave those people who had actually been victimized a score of six or higher on a scale of one to ten to show vulnerability. The study showed that inmates with a violent criminal past chose their victims based on gait—how they walked.

What does this mean to the average person? *The way you carry yourself can help single you out, or rule you out, as a target for violent criminals.* While there are victim selection criteria like your gender or age that you have no control over, you can change the way you are perceived by violent offenders. Walking confidently, head up, shoulders back, and not succumbing to distractions (like having your head buried in your cellphone) are easy ways to help minimize your chances of being singled out as a target.

In the simplest terms, do you walk like you have the ability to defend yourself? Or, do you drag your feet and act like a wounded animal, being targeted by the wolves who want to do you harm? While you cannot control the people around you or their depravity, you can control your image and whether or not you carry yourself like a victim.

Along this same principle is having a good sense of what is happening around you. In the world of special agents, operators, and warriors we call this "keeping your head on a swivel" and having good "Situational Awareness."

Situational Awareness Defined

As the names implies, situational awareness is simply knowing what's going on around you. It sounds easy in principle, but in reality it requires practice. This skill is ingrained in special agents, soldiers, law enforcement officers, and government-trained operatives. It is also a critical skill for civilians as well. Ultimately, being aware of a threat, even seconds before everyone else, can keep you and your loved ones safe.

Situational awareness is a skill that can and should be developed for reasons outside personal defense and safety. Situational awareness is really just another word for mindfulness. Developing this awareness has allowed me to survive multiple overseas operations in very high-threat environments, and to be more cognizant of what's happening around me in my daily activities. Although the focus is primarily on developing one's situational awareness to prevent or recognize a violent attack *before* it happens, it has also helped me make better decisions in all aspects of my life.

Research on situational awareness indicates it can be cultivated by generally keeping tabs on your surroundings—"checking your six" (watching or observing what is behind you), "head on a swivel," and "keeping your back to the wall."

That's exactly what situational awareness is: knowing what's going on by scanning your environment. But what it doesn't do is tell me, "What exactly am I looking for? How do I know if I'm paying attention to (observing) the right things? Are there behaviors (pre-incident indicators) or warning signs of an imminent threat that I should be aware of?"

In order to understand situational awareness, you must first understand the OODA loop process.

How to Reset Your Opponent's OODA Loop

Wikipedia defines the OODA loop as an acronym for **observe, orient, decide**, and **act**. It was developed by military strategist and US Air Force Colonel John Boyd. Boyd first applied the concept to aerial combat (dog fighting) during the 1950s.

His approach favors agility over raw power when dealing with human opponents in any endeavor. The OODA loop is a process we go through hundreds, if not thousands, of times each day. It is a process that defines how humans react to stimuli. Colonel Boyd believed you can overcome a disadvantage by attacking the mind of your opponent. Attacking the mind, or resetting your opponent's OODA loop, could be anything from moving, a loud noise, a slap in the face, or anything that causes your opponent to re-observe, re-orient, re-decide, and re-act to your stimuli. Thus, providing you more time to complete your action. The person who can cycle through the OODA loop the fastest, wins—whether it's running away, drawing your weapon, or attacking your opponent.

Remember my story in the previous chapter where I described the incident in the Inner Harbor of Baltimore? The reason my actions worked—making eye contact; raising my hand high; saying, "How are you guys doing? Good to see you again!"— was because I upset those two men's OODA loop process. I disrupted and altered their decision-making process (their OODA loop) long enough to walk away from their inner space, where they wanted to engage in a potentially violent confrontation. This buys you time to escape or force the bad guy to: re-observe, re-orient, re-decide, and re-act from his original intention.

Here's another scenario: You are walking along a quiet street at night and a person comes around the corner who immediately spikes your "gift of fear." Your intuition tells you something is not right about this person, but you have no other option but to continue along in your direction of travel. So first, raise your hand high above your shoulder. This action will make you look bigger (it is the reason a bear rears up on its hinds legs prior to an attack); it will also cause your would-be assailant to avert his eyes to your raised hand. With his eyes looking at your raised hand, you use your other hand to prepare to draw your weapon (tactical pen, keys, handgun).

At the same time, as he approaches, you look him straight in the eye, with a big smile on your face and say, "How are you doing tonight? Good to see you again," as you continue your direct path to the nearest area where there are other people around. As human beings, we are programmed to answer a question posed to us. By asking, "How are you doing tonight?" causes a disruption in the attackers OODA loop process. He is processing how to respond to your direct question. By stating, "Good to see you again," you are totally disrupting and altering his OODA loop process once again. The would-be attacker is now wondering how you know him. His OODA loop is now completely offtrack, and this should buy you time to walk past him as he considers other options.

Another "trick" to alter someone's OODA loop when your gut is telling you something is not quite right, is to let out a loud "whoop-whoop" and scream, "Purple Unicorn!" This will not only attract the attention of others nearby, but it will completely reset your would-be assailant's OODA loop. He may think you are completely crazy. But who cares? He is a stranger after all. You would be surprised how effective this technique truly is. By letting out a big "whoop" or scream, followed by "pink flying monkeys" or anything that sounds completely out of context, yelled at the top of your voice, is a very effective way to make your would-be assailant look for another victim. Your assailant may think you are insane. That's okay, in my thirty-one years in law enforcement I have learned even criminals do not want to mess with "crazy."

I have a former client who told me a story of how she was able to thwart a certain attack by using the OODA loop to her advantage. My client, a woman in her mid-thirties, was jogging on a bike path around the lake in our neighborhood one evening. As she rounded a sharp turn, she noticed a man lurking in the tree line. As she passed him, she greeted him with a smile and a "good evening." She admitted her intuition immediately told her something was not right. She picked up her pace and quickly noticed he started running after her. When she approached the nearest clearing, she ran to a grassy area along the path, got down on all fours, started barking like a dog and eating grass.

This may sound like a crazy woman or even a crazy idea, but her quick actions and innovative idea probably saved her life. The man stopped running. My client said she saw him shake his head in wonder, and run in the other direction, back into the tree line. Her quick thinking certainly reset her would-be attacker's OODA loop. He may have thought she was crazy, but this woman surely outsmarted and outplayed her assailant's OODA loop process.

The action of an individual who can process through the OODA cycle quickly—observing and reacting to unfolding events—gains the advantage. In every course I teach, I use this decision cycle. I am constantly teaching my clients that in order to survive you must move, by moving you are upsetting your opponents OODA loop process, buying time to get off the X and removing yourself from a critical situation.

Most people associate situational awareness with the first step in the cycle—observe. But it's the second step in the OODA loop—orient—that answers the questions about what developing situational awareness actually involves. Orientation tells us what we should look for when we are observing, then puts those observations into context so we know what to do with the information.

Observe + Orient = Situational Awareness

How to "Live in the Yellow"

How can we become better observers in order to improve our situational awareness? And how should we orient ourselves so that we observe the right things and understand the context of what we're seeing?

In *Principles of Personal Defense* (1989), gun-fighting expert Jeff Cooper devised **a color-code system to help measure a person's mindset for combat scenarios** (see chart below). Each color represents a person's potential state of awareness and focus.

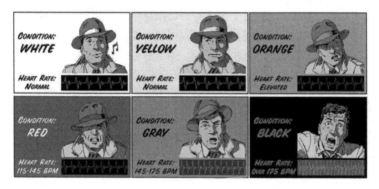

Figure 1 Cooper Situational Awareness Color Codes

For optimal situational awareness, you want to stay in Condition Yellow—that is, "Live in the Yellow!"

Condition Yellow is best described as "relaxed alert." There's no specific threat situation, but you have your head up and you're observing your surroundings with all your senses. Most people associate situational awareness with just using vision—looking at one's environment. But you want to use all of your senses when assessing your situation and environment. You can learn a lot from the sounds (or lack thereof) and even the smells in an environment.

Even though your senses are slightly heightened in Condition Yellow, it's also important to stay relaxed. By adopting a calm demeanor, you won't bring any unnecessary attention to yourself. If you look nervous, or you're overtly "checking your six" with your head swiveling frantically while you scan your surroundings, people are going to notice you. Additionally, staying relaxed ensures that you maintain an open focus, which allows you to take in more information about what's going on around you. Research shows that when we get nervous or stressed, our attention narrows, causing us to concentrate on just a few things at a time—tunnel vision and selected hearing. A narrow focus can cause us to miss important details in our environment.

Try to avoid Condition White (being unaware) when you are at work or in public places. As I often say in my training courses, "Don't walk around as if everything is rainbows and unicorns." Make Condition Yellow a habit. When you observe a potential pre-incident indicator, or you notice something that isn't the "norm" for the environment, or if your Gift of Fear starts speaking to you, quickly analyze the situation and take the appropriate action.

Throughout the day, strive to have good situational awareness or Condition Yellow. If you identify potential dangers, switch to Condition Orange and apply the OODA loop. In the rare instances that require an immediate response, switch to Condition Red. Switch back to Condition Yellow after the threat has been resolved. Repeat this exercise and situational awareness will become habit. Condition Black is being so stressed with a pulse rate so high that you are virtually unresponsive to the threat—you're "frozen in fear." Freezing in any critical event or crisis situation is a mistake that often leads to serious injury or death.

Bottom line: Look up from your smartphone; don't zone out; open your eyes, ears, and nose; and calmly scan your environment to take in what's going on around you. Also, don't wear headphones—you lose environmental awareness. When you take away your sense of hearing, you have essentially handicapped yourself before an assailant even enters the picture. Without your sense of hearing, you're a prime target for mugging, sexual assault, and any other crime that relies on the element of surprise.

In addition to "Living in the Yellow," use these additional skills to improve your observational abilities: Put yourself in a position where you can best observe your surroundings. In order to gain your situational awareness, you need to be able to see, hear and smell as much of your surroundings as possible. Positioning yourself in obstructed spots will inhibit the flow of information you're trying to collect. So whenever you enter a new environment, put yourself in a position that will allow you to see as much as possible, without being surprised from behind. I recommend finding a place where you can view all or most of the entrance points that also allows you to put your back to the wall. This position enables you to

- see who enters your environment;
- identify all the exits and readies you to make a quick getaway; and
- eliminate the possibility of failing to see a threat materialize behind you.

This isn't possible in all situations. You can't always control which table a restaurant hostess will seat you on a busy night, and you would likely get a lot of strange looks if you stood with your back in a corner while you're waiting for your order at McDonald's. So do your best within the given circumstances. In that busy restaurant, you might not have control of your table location, but you can choose which seat you take. Pick the chair that gives you the best view from your table. When you're standing in line at a fast food restaurant, nonchalantly look around and take in the scene.

I-Spy Game

Hone your observation skills by playing the "I-Spy Game." I used to play it with my kids and now my grandkids. This I-Spy game has a bit of a twist and helps to develop your situational awareness and strengthens your observational skills. The game is simple. When you go into a business, make a mental note of a few things about the environment: How many workers are behind the counter? What are people wearing? How many exits are there? Is there an AED or fire extinguisher in the room? When you head home, ask your kids' questions like, "I spied with my eye, a fire extinguisher. Where was it?" Or, "I spied with my eye, a Yankees baseball cap. Who was wearing it? What color was his shirt?" You get the idea.

It is fun to play, but more importantly it's training your kids to be more mindful of their surroundings.

Being more observant isn't enough to master situational awareness. You have to know what you're looking for, then put that information into context so it has meaning and becomes actionable. That's where the *Orient* phase comes into play.

The orient step provides three things to help us achieve situational awareness:

1. Establishes and identifies **baselines** and **anomalies** for our particular environment.
2. Identifies certain models of human behavior we should look for (e.g., **watch the hands** and **act natural**).
3. Develops a **plan of action** depending on our observations.

Establish a Baseline Wherever You Go

Every environment and person has a baseline. A baseline is the "normal" in any given situation. It will differ from person to person and environment to environment. For example, the baseline at a small coffee shop will usually entail people reading books or working on their computers or speaking in hushed tones with their friends. The baseline at a movie theater would be people standing in line to buy popcorn, waiting outside the restroom for their dates, or checking the status board for the time and location of the movie they want to see.

What about the baseline at your home? By establishing baselines at your house, you will be able to immediately sense when something is not right. Have you ever returned home and found the garage door open? Did you assume you had just forgotten to close it as you left? Or, did you recognize this was not the "norm" and took appropriate action and had either the police or a neighbor assist you in making sure your home was empty and safe?

We establish baselines so that we can spot anomalies. According to situational awareness expert Patrick Van Horne, an instructor of the Marine Combat Profiling system, and author of *Left of Bang* (2014), "anomalies are things that either do not happen and should, or that do happen and shouldn't." Anomalies are what grab our attention as we take in our surroundings and what we need to focus on to achieve situational awareness.

The first step in orienting ourselves is to establish baselines so that we can direct our attention to anomalies. It's actually quite simple. Every time you enter a new environment, you mentally ask yourself these two sets of questions:

- **Baseline Questions:** What's going on here? What's the general mood of the place? What is the "normal" activity that I should expect here? How do most people behave here most of the time?
- **Anomaly Questions:** What would cause someone or something to stand out? What would be "abnormal" for this particular environment?

For instance, if you were to enter the lobby of a movie theater and notice a man standing alone in the corner, with his back against the wall and his hands in his pockets, this should stand out to you as something that is out of the norm for a moviegoer. He may be totally innocent and a nonthreat. But his positioning

and out of the norm behavior is not what you'd expect for someone in a movie theater and this should raise your suspicion.
Those that are in tune with the baseline of their surroundings
are able to pick up on the subtle clues that something is wrong.
These people not only understand what a baseline should look
like, but they are also not letting their rationalization cloud their
view.

Our inability to pay attention to everything all at once makes
it impossible to obtain complete situational awareness. The
human mind can only take in so much information at any given
time. Therefore, in regards to our personal safety, where things
unfold quickly and seconds are often the difference between life
and death, how we direct our attention is paramount.

Think about a bus or a subway ride—passengers generally
appear pretty relaxed while they stare out the window or read
a book. Some even fall asleep (please do not do that on public
transportation; it provides you absolutely zero situational awareness). If someone looks uncomfortable, that's an anomaly that
warrants extra attention, but it does not necessarily mean they're
a threat. They could be distressed because they are late for work
or maybe they are under financial stress. Again, it's just something to keep your eye on.

A common display of uncomfortable behavior that you may
see in someone who is up to no good is constantly "checking
their six." This is when a person continually looks over their
shoulder to see what is behind them. People who are comfortable generally don't do this because they don't feel any threat.
Now obviously, "checking your six" is something that situationally aware good guys do too. However, if you're doing it right, it
should not be noticeable to others, but it takes practice. So if you
see a guy continually looking over his shoulder when he should
be standing there unconcerned, that's an anomaly that should
get your attention and raise your suspicion.

On the flipside, someone acting comfortable when everyone else is uncomfortable would be an anomaly. One of the ways law enforcement was able to identify the Boston Marathon bombers was they noticed in surveillance footage that two men looked relatively calm while everyone else was running around in a panic. The reason these two men looked so calm admid the chaos was because they were the ones who built and placed the bombs. Having foreknowledge of the explosion allowed them to calmly walk the streets of Boston while those around them were scurrying looking for safety.

Another measure of suspicion is noticing how interested or uninterested someone's behavior may be. Most people are not paying attention to their environment. They are too caught up in their own thoughts or whatever they're doing. So individuals who are showing interest in a particular person or object that most people wouldn't be interested in, is an anomaly that warrants further observation. For instance, if you're sitting at an outdoor café and you notice the person sitting a few tables away staring at the entrance to the building across the street. The person is just sitting there, maybe with a cup of coffee on the table, seemingly overly interested in the building across the street. This behavior does not match the "norm" for the environment at an outdoor café and this should capture your attention. Again, maybe this person is looking for his friend to come out of the building, or maybe he has more devious plans. Either way, his abnormal behavior for the environment should have been noticed if you're maintaining good situational awareness.

These body language identifiers establish baselines for every situation and allow us to direct our attention toward things that are potentially a threat. If a person's behavior fits the baseline for that particular environment or circumstance, you can ignore them. If their behavior doesn't fit the baseline, they're an anomaly and you should observe them more closely.

Look for certain models of human behavior.

Here are few other Behavioral Threat Indicators to look for:

First, checking the hands of a suspicious person ensures that the person is not holding a weapon and is not preparing to strike. Secondly, individuals concealing a weapon such as a gun or knife will often touch or pat that area on the body where the weapon is concealed. They unconsciously do this to ensure the object has not been lost or is still hidden from view.

Second, act natural. It's difficult to "act natural" when you are involved in criminal activity or planning an attack. People "acting" natural will appear "un-natural" and will often over or under-exaggerate their movements. Look for these movements which you will recognize as being *abnormal for the environment* and maintain your vigilance.

Have a plan of action based on what you observe.

Say you decide to stop in at your local Starbucks and a bad guy decides to visit at the same time to rob the establishment and everyone present, including you. But because you've followed the principles above, you noticed him and recognized him as a threat when he walked in. You observed the fact that he did not meet the baseline for Starbucks, and as an anomaly, you recognized the need to act.

Great. Now what?

Seconds matter. You do not have time to formulate a well-thought-out plan of action. What's more, the stress of the event will muddle your thinking and decision-making process. In addition to asking yourself the baseline and anomaly questions every time you enter an environment, ask yourself a third question: What would I do if I saw an anomaly? In other words, come up with an action plan.

So let's go back to the Starbucks example. The anomaly for which you want to create an action plan is "a guy comes in with a gun." The best course of action in this scenario depends on a few things, as well as you being situationally aware. If the robber came in from the front door, and you're near the rear exit, your best action would be to **get off the X** and run out the back door as fast as you can. On the other hand, if he entered through the back exit near you, your best course of action would be to either run past him, or through him, as fast and hard as you can. If you cannot escape, you can shelter-in-place in the restroom. Most Starbucks locations have concrete walls, steel door frames, steel doors, and a sturdy lock, which makes for a great room to retreat if you cannot get of the X.

Situational awareness is a mindset that you have to purposefully cultivate. You want to get to the point that it's just something you do without having to think about it. To get there, you have to practice it regularly. Starting today, consciously remind yourself to look for exit points whenever you enter a new building. Start observing people and establishing baselines and generating possible anomalies while you're at home, school, work, at the gym, or on a date. Then, start thinking about action plans on what you would do in a specific situation. Don't be paranoid, just be aware and mindful. Don't be afraid, be ready. Do that day in and day out, and situational awareness won't be something you have to intentionally think about, it will just be.

Anything we can do to be more alert and aware makes us less likely to become a target. So, establish baselines. Look for anomalies. Always have a plan. Live in the Yellow. That's what defines good Situational Awareness.

Effective Strikes: Eyes, Throat, Knees

The only fight you are 100 percent sure to win is the one you never get into. In a fight, everyone gets hurt—everyone. Without hesitation I will tell you, avoid every fight possible. The only time to engage in a fight is when it is the only option available, and your safety and well-being are at risk.

Street fighting is often glamorized in films and TV shows but in real-life, it is a very dangerous situation as you never know the mindset or skill set of your adversary. There are simply far too many factors and too many unknowns that can go wrong in a fight. Even the most skilled martial artists know not to engage, unless they have no other choice or when it is solely a self-defense type situation.

That being said, if you do have to strike—strike first and strike with a vengeance. You are not trying to injure or hurt your adversary; you are trying to incapacitate and destroy your enemy so you can escape with your life. Tim Larkin states in *When Violence is the Answer* (2017), "Violence isn't chess at ninety miles per hour. It's demolition derby. And just like demolition derby, it's the driver with the most forward momentum who usually wins."

A perennial favorite is the **eye gouge** and it's exactly what it sounds like. Either two fingers are thrust into the eyes sockets or two thumbs. The fingers are aimed to slide in under the eyeballs, while the thumbs should be aimed for the inner corners of the eye, near the nose. Either way, the goal is to scoop the eyes out or crush them inside the occipital cavity. The eyes are the most vulnerable area on every mammal on earth. Destroy the eyes and you will have destroyed your enemy.

The **throat punch** isn't just a common internet joke. The Marine Corps lists the throat as a good target for both lead-hand punches and rear-hand punches. A good strike to the throat can crush the windpipe, while a more modest strike is certainly going to cause pain and throw your opponent off balance. Go straight for the Adam's apple and remember to follow through with your strike. That is, punch (or strike) through your opponent—envision yourself striking the target area and driving through it an additional three feet.

A four-finger strike, with your fingers aimed directly at the soft area of the throat, located below the Adam's apple, is also an effective strike which will incapacitate your enemy. Again, if you do this, strike without hesitation and with a 100 percent commitment to stop, neutralize, and to destroy your attacker's will to continue.

> "Give me the biggest guy in the world, you
> smash his **knee** and he'll drop like a stone"
> —Patrick Swayze, from the cult classic film *Roadhouse*

Patrick Swayze was right; **the knee** is a very vulnerable target to strike. There is a reason why there are severe penalties in football, hockey, soccer and even the MMA (Mixed Martial Arts) when it comes to attacking the knee. It you are able to destroy your adversary's knee with a strong kick, it could provide you the opportunity to escape.

Any **elbow strike** can do some damage. The elbow is the hardest part of your body—use it often in a fight. There's the low-to-high blow that strikes an enemy beneath the chin, the horizontal blow that smashes into a soft spot of the body or face, and then there's striking an enemy on the base of the skull as he is bent or doubled over. The elbow is an effective weapon.

The **"Double Palm Strike"** is a blow that holds power to do extensive damage. Put palm over palm and drive your hands as hard as you can into the unsuspecting attacker's face. This should provide you an opportunity to escape as your adversary crumbles to the floor.

There is no substitute for inflicting debilitating injury. It turns a life-or-death situation in your favor. It makes a large, strong, scary man into an injured man helpless to keep you from escaping or delivering a final blow.

As you learned in the first chapter, Survival Mindset, if violence is the last resort, you better be good at it! If you are going to have to use an incapacitating strike in order to save your life, do so with all the strength, power, commitment, and determination your body can muster. In a fight for your life, there is no substitute for inflicting the greatest amount of injury on your attacker. Violence is a tool, and when violence is the answer, that is, it is the only thing that will save your life—it is the only answer! Those who survive violent encounters do so because they have the mindset and the intent to do real harm (injury) to another human-being when real harm is what's required. If you fail to be effective with your strike because you hesitated or had a second of doubt, it may very well be the last act of your life.

Teaching Situational Awareness to Your Children

I've already discussed how to hone your observation skills and that of your children by playing the "I-Spy Game." It is fun to play, but more importantly it's training them to be more mindful of their surroundings.

Code Word

A "code word" is used to communicate to your family, or others in your inner circle that danger is imminent and everyone should leave the area immediately—without argument, without question, without trying to see what is happening. When the code word is uttered, everyone must evacuate the area immediately. Once in a safe place, call 911 and advise the authorities.

In my family, we use the word "wildfire." My children have known from a very early age that if I ever said the word "wildfire," they would move without question. The technique works like this: Suppose you're at a restaurant for a family dinner when you notice two men walk in the front door. The two men instantly spike your "gift of fear." Your gut instinct and intuition are screaming at you that something about those two men is not right. You observed them when they entered the restaurant because you chose your seat wisely and you are using good situational awareness. You have visited this restaurant before and have established a "baseline" for what is normal—and these two men do not meet the normal standard. Maybe they look uncomfortable when everyone else seems at ease. Maybe they are constantly "checking their six," or their hands are buried deep in their pockets—things that are setting off alarms that something is not right!

You lean across the table and tell your wife and kids, "Wildfire! Wildfire! Wildfire!" You all immediately stand up and exit the restaurant as quickly as you can without bringing attention to yourself. If you have already ordered, you can always return to pay the bill later. If you ignore your gut instinct, you may find yourself in an armed robbery or hostage situation. If you leave and nothing happens, no harm is done and you've provided your kids with a great story to tell and you've shown them the importance of listening to your inner voice. I think a little embarrassment is far better than ignoring your instincts and putting your family's lives at risk.

Sit down with your family and create a code word or short phrase that is easy to remember, but one not used in everyday conversation. A word that says, "DANGER, LEAVE NOW!" I hope you never have to use your code word, but **it's better to have it and not need it than need it and not have it.**

Duress Word

Another word to develop within your family is a "duress word." This word will be used in communication with your loved ones if a situation occurs where you can't speak freely or are under someone else's control. For instance, if you were kidnapped and held at gunpoint, you would use your duress word in the conversation to signal help is needed.

I will address other ideas on how to keep your children safe in the "Home Security" chapter.

Chapter 3
YOUR EDC (EVERYDAY CARRY)

What does the term "everyday carry" mean? In the literal sense, your everyday carry (EDC) is the collection of items you carry with you in your pockets or in your purse on a daily basis that may be of assistance to you in a critical situation.

They're the things you tap your pockets for before you head out the door; the things you feel naked without, and the things that would throw off your whole day if you had to do without them. They are not especially valuable, but consist of items that you find truly essential.

The everyday carry philosophy is built upon the cornerstones of functionality and preparedness. Each component of your EDC should serve a purpose and have at least one, if not several, specific functions. Your EDC items prepare you for the worst and empower you to do your best.

I wish I could say the FBI had its own version of "Q"—the famous James Bond movie character that provided the suave, sophisticated, and tactically skilled British Secret Agent with all the toys any man would ever want. Unfortunately, they do not; and my wrist-watch does not have a laser that cuts through steel, nor do my shoes have removable heels that explode when thrown, and my ring doesn't have a secret camera. So, I have to choose what I carry – things that are versatile, lightweight, and will help me in numerous situations. Of course, these EDC items are in addition to the three items almost everyone carries—their cell phone, wallet, and keys.

Remember this:

The "will to survive" (Survival Mindset)
is the best tool you have,

but EDC tools also help!

Three Must-Have Items

Everyone has their own idea of what should be carried and why. In my thirty years of being security conscious, no matter where I travel, I have come up with these three must-have items:

Tactical Pen

A tactical pen is one of my all-time favorite personal defense tools. It is versatile, compact, affordable and functional. In addition, you can take it anywhere. I've carried mine into court houses, airplanes, and sporting events. Usually designed from aircraft-grade aluminum, they generally write very well, but they can be used as a potent weapon in a crisis situation. Many have a tungsten steel glass-breaking tip, which could be used to break a window in an emergency situation, such as your car slowly submerging under water.

The tactical pen is also the weapon I carry when I go running. It easily clips onto my shirt or running shorts, or I can just carry it in my hand, where it's mostly concealed and ready for use against an attack from a man or vicious dog. In my training courses, I always recommend everyone purchase and carry a tactical pen. A strike to the face, eyes, or throat with this pen will incapacitate most assailants. A quick stab to the hands, forearms, thigh, or groin would certainly make them release their grip and afford you the opportunity to run and escape.

You can purchase a tactical pen in almost any gun store and certainly on Amazon. My favorite is the Smith & Wesson 6.1-inch aircraft aluminum tactical pull-cap pen.

Flashlight

Chances are you would carry an umbrella if the weather forecast called for a 50 percent chance of rain, so why wouldn't you bring a flashlight for 100 percent chance of darkness every night? From getting through power outages, to looking under couches, to navigating a dimly lit path, having a light source in your pocket will come in handy. Some might be content with using their cell phone's screen for light, however, modern flashlights, with multiple modes and a dedicated battery, perform far better and will not drain your phone's battery. A good flashlight is a must-have whenever I leave the house.

Another reason for carrying a good tactical flashlight is it prevents you from not looking like a victim. Having a flashlight allows you to better observe in the darkness, but it can also act as a deterrent to would-be assailants. At night, law enforcement officers are usually the only ones shining flashlights down alleys and dark places. Therefore, if you're shining your light as you walk to your destination or back to your car, the bad guys may think you're a cop and will look for another victim. If you are confronted by an assailant, you can use the tactical flashlight as a defensive tool by blinding your attacker with the bright beam or hitting him with the beveled edge that's often built into the end.

The size of flashlights and their lumen (brightness of their beam) varies greatly. You should have a small, yet powerful, flashlight that fits into your pocket or onto your key chain; and you should have a second bigger, brighter, beveled edged, tactical flashlight in your purse, briefcase, or backpack.

Multi-tool

The multi-tool embodies many core principles of EDC—utility, versatility, and portability. For quick fixes, tinkering, and other handy work, having a single tool that fits easily into your pocket is invaluable. Common multi-tool functions include pliers, screwdrivers, bottle openers, scissors, and other cutting tools. These multi-tools also come in a variety of sizes, not all of which are meant for EDC. Choose one that meets your needs and carry it with you wherever you go.

Is it absolutely necessary to carry all this stuff? Not at all. Everyday carry is all about creating a setup that fits your lifestyle. Just as no two people are exactly alike, their respective EDCs will vary significantly. Acquire and carry what you need according to your lifestyle, location, profession, daily routine, budget, and so on. This is especially true if you want to carry a firearm or a knife. I carry both whenever I leave home. However, if I am traveling by air or traveling internationally, I am limited in what I can carry. There are numerous restrictions and stiff penalties for illegally carrying weapons. It's your responsibility to be well-informed and know what local laws require. Be sure to do your due diligence before traveling with a gun or knife.

EDC with a Backpack, Shoulder Bag, or Laptop Bag

My flashlight, multi-tool, and tactical pen are always on my person, that is, in my pocket, clipped to my belt, or in the breast pocket of my suit. If I know I am going somewhere where a backpack is appropriate, then I carry that over my shoulder as well. This back pack, if not carried on me, is always with me in the back seat of my truck under a blanket or coat—readily available. The reason I have a backpack with all the "essentials" to survive a crisis situation is based on an old Warrior code:

"Better to have it and not need it; than need it and not have it."

The backpack acts as my secondary EDC personal protection gear. Obviously I can carry much more in a small, lightweight backpack than in my pockets. If I know I will be conducting business on my computer, I can quickly and easily move my backpack items into a laptop bag. Either way, the following items are usually within reach, and I recommend you develop your own list of items you feel you would need in a critical situation or high-threat environment. My backpack contains the following:

Spare Ammunition and Spare Magazines
I carry a box of fifty rounds plus two fully loaded, spare magazines (to be discussed in a later chapter).

A Good Knife
Many everyday carry lists include a pocket knife. I always have a knife clipped to my right pants pocket. While the laws on blade length differ in each state, a well-designed, reasonably sized pocketknife is primarily a tool. When used responsibly, a knife safely handles cutting and slicing tasks—usually better than a house key, a pair of scissors, or your hands. With that said, not everyone is skilled with a knife, or even legally allowed to carry one. But it's important to view them for their practicality. Although I "everyday carry" a three-inch folding knife on my person, I also have a larger, more functional five-inch fixed-blade knife in my backpack.

As a testament that we are never too old to learn, in a recent training I learned the value of a fixed blade versus a folding blade knife. It is virtually impossible in the middle of a fight, to extract your folding knife from your pocket or clipped to your belt, open the blade, and use it to defend yourself. However, if you have a fixed-blade in a scabbard, attached to your body (the number of concealed carry options is unlimited), drawing the blade in the heat, stress, and violence of a fight is fairly easy and is a great way to end the fight. Lesson learned—a fixed-blade knife is a better option than a folding blade for everyday carry.

Medical

I always have a small medical bag in my backpack that contains:

- **C.A.T. (Combat Application Tourniquet)** or **R.A.T.S. (Rapid Application Tourniquet System) tourniquet:** This one-handed tourniquet system is known to be the best response for serious bleeding from a limb. Tourniquets have saved thousands of lives in both Afghanistan and Iraq.
- **QuikClot:** A gauze bandage that is coated with a unique substance that accelerates your body's natural clotting process. Both the QuikClot and the CAT tourniquet are always with me when I'm teaching a firearms course. Note: I have never had to use this during any of my training courses!
- **Minor Injury Treatment:** Bandages, Band-Aids, alcohol swabs, mole skin, hydrocortisone (anti-itch), Benadryl (for allergic reactions), aspirin (for pain and heart attacks), ipecac (to induce vomiting), 4x4 gauzes, steri-strips, etc. I always have a Med-Kit close at hand, in my backpack, truck, Go-Bag, and in my home.

Waterproof & Windproof Matches

I store these in a hard, dry container. You never know when you're going to need a fire for warmth, to signal, or to destroy.

Fire Source

I use cotton balls dipped in Petroleum Jelly. This is my "fire starter." If you take your basic cotton ball and dip it in petroleum jelly you have an instant way to start a fire with just a spark. The cotton ball will burn for two to three minutes and allow you to add kindling or a primary burning source. I store ten to twelve "Vaseline" dipped cotton balls in an old 35mm film container, but any small, waterproof container such as a plastic pill bottle will work. These petroleum jelly-laced cotton balls will last for years.

Light Source (Flashlight)

I carry both a headlamp for hands-free light and an extra tactical flashlight with a beveled edge in my backpack. I also carry spare batteries for both; however, in the Texas summer heat these batteries will drain very quickly.

550 Cord / ParaCord (10 feet)

There are many uses for paracord. You may need to tie something up to keep if off the floor; or tie something down to prevent it from blowing away. It can be used to replace a broken shoe lace and be used to get out of restraints—to be discussed in a later chapter.

Duct Tape (10 feet)

Wrap the duct tape around a small pencil. I believe in the old saying, "If you can't fix it with duct tape, it can't be fixed." That may not be entirely true, but a lot of items can be fixed with this versatile product. There are dozens of websites and YouTube videos detailing the many uses of duct tape. The most common uses include fixing a leak, whether it's on a window, a pipe, a tent, or a cup. It also comes in handy if you need to secure items together.

Large Multi-Tool

As previously discussed in my EDC, this multi-tool embodies utility, versatility, and portability. I carry a small one in my pocket, and a much larger one in my backpack. It's like carrying ten tools in one. You will be surprised how often you use this tool once you make a habit of always having one nearby.

Metal Water Bottle

A small, liter sized, metal water bottle can always be found in the side pouch of my backpack. Water is the source of life— always have some with you. It quenches thirst, cleans wounds, and cools you down.

Travel Toothbrush & Toothpaste

Hygiene is important even during a crisis. Besides, you never know when someone is going to sneak onions onto your sandwich just before you're meeting with an important client.

Weatherproof Writing Pad such as "Rain Writer"

Having a pen and paper handy is critical for leaving notes, jotting down important numbers, documenting critical information, or sketching out an Operations Plan.

Extra Tactical Pen

If you're going to have a writing tablet, you're going to need a pen. If you're going to need a pen, it might as well be a good tactical pen. I like to think you can never have too many improvised weapons!

Handcuffs and Flex Cuffs

Obviously great for securing people, but also good for securing items. It's become a force of habit for me to always have restraints readily available. I feel at risk if I don't have a means of securing a bad guy.

Chem-Lights

These are good for additional lighting and can also be used to identify your location, mark your trail, communicate a hazard, or keep track of moving items or people. It's a great alternate light source without using heat or requiring a spark or battery. They last for hours and can be used indoors or out. They're not affected by temperature or the wind, they will work in or near water, come in a variety of colors (and infrared), they're inexpensive and are ideal in hazardous environments such as gas leaks or noxious fumes. It's like having a candle without a flame! If you're not familiar with Chem-Lights, they are also known as glow sticks and are a form of chemical lighting. They are made with a plastic sheath or tube that houses a mixture of chemicals. The way it works is you bend the sheath (outer tube) to crack the inner capsule, located inside the tube. Once you break the inner capsule, you shake it up to mix the contents, creating a chemical reaction that emits light with only a miniscule emission of heat. I always have six or eight of these in my backpack and scattered throughout my truck.

Small Binoculars

When you see something off in the distance and you want or need to know what it is, having a nice pair of binoculars available is essential. I carry a small pair in my backpack and a larger, more powerful pair in my "Go-Bag" (to be discussed later in this chapter).

Magnetic Compass

In crisis situations, it's always good to know which direction you're going and how to get there!

Navy Blue or Nondescript Baseball Hat

Having a hat available is important to contain your body heat, keep the sun off your head, protect you from rain and snow, and to alter or conceal your identity if needed.

A Few "Tradecraft" Skills

In addition to my EDC and my backpack, I have some recommendations for items to carry that I have learned over the years, which could make a difference in a crisis or high-threat environment:

Handcuff Keys

I always have a handcuff key duct-taped to the inside of my belt at the small of my back. In addition, I have a key on every key chain and several in my car, backpack, and Go-Bag. You never know when having a handcuff key might be useful. Since I always have a set of handcuffs in my backpack, it makes sense to have an extra key readily available. You should know that handcuff keys are NOT restricted by TSA and will be allowed on aircraft. I advise all my clients who travel overseas to tape a key to the inside of their belts, in their shoes, or secreted in their jackets.

Hair Barrettes/Hair Clips

These are easy to conceal and can be used to get you out of handcuffs (I will teach you this trick in a later chapter). Just slip one or two over the top of your pants along your waist. Or keep one in your ball cap if you routinely wear hats. Or if you have long hair, put one under your hair, along the back of your neck. These are cheap, light, easily hidden and a must-carry item if you're traveling overseas.

Go Bags

The world is an unpredictable place. You don't have to look far to see that having the right attitude, the right knowledge, and the right tools can make the difference between life and death. Accidents, weather, natural disasters, disease, civil unrest, and violence can instantly alter our safe, secure world and plunge us into danger.

You never know where or when you're going to be faced with a critical, life-or-death situation. Could you and your family survive in your own home should you be trapped and unable to get food or water? How long could you survive if something goes horribly wrong while you are out for a drive?

There are hundreds of examples of people and families being stranded because their vehicle broke down in the middle of the desert, or they drove off the highway in a blinding blizzard and encased their vehicle in a snowbank, or due to natural disaster they become trapped in their own home for days before help can arrive. Having a Go-Bag is one way of surviving these types of ordeals.

A Go-Bag is different than an EDC Backpack in that the Go-Bag is primarily used for emergency evacuation in times of natural disaster or in a serious crisis. In preparing your Go-Bag, you should pack items that will allow you to survive without assistance for three to four days. This bag should be something you take with you if you're traveling on vacation, a long road-trip, or when visiting relatives across state lines.

Begin by buying a good bag for everyone in your household. The bag should be a backpack made with water resistant material and able to be closed to keep items dry. Each member of your household should have their own bag. Suitcases should not be considered, as they are bulky, clumsy, and difficult to carry except on smooth surfaces. Once the bags are packed they should all be placed in one location where everyone knows to grab all the bags in the event of a critical situation that requires evacuation.

Documents

Next you need to scan all of your important, personal documents and save it both on a thumb drive and in the cloud, including:

- Driver's License
- Passport
- Deed to Your Home
- Birth Certificates
- Your Will or Trust
- Social Security Card
- Medical Records
- List of Medications
- Contact Telephone Numbers & Addresses
- Proof of Insurance—Auto, Life, Home
- Bank Accounts & Credit Cards

Also, take a photo of every room in your home focusing on high-value items and save those in the cloud, on your memory stick, and if possible on your cell phone.

Pack water and canned food or camping-style food: Put two liters of water in each family member's backpack and enough food or snacks to sustain each person for 72 hours (that is not a lot of food). Remember, you can survive weeks without food—but only days without water. Military-style MREs (Meals Ready-to-Eat) are ideal as they contain a high caloric and high protein count. One MRE is designed to be able to sustain a soldier for the entire day. Three to four MRE packs take up little space in your Go-Bag.

Also include some energy bars, preferably those not containing materials that can melt (chocolate), and be sure they are packaged in waterproof wrappers.

Clothes

The environment where you live determines what type of clothing you want to pack. But remember, you may have to travel a great distance (for example, in a hurricane evacuation) to be safe and the weather patterns can change rapidly within just a few hours drive. I recommend:

- Blue jeans or cargo pants (1 pair)
- Underwear (2 pair)
- Socks (Smart Wool makes a great all-weather sock, 2 pair)
- Tee shirt (preferably a Dry-Fit, or moisture wicking material
- Button-down shirt
- Fleece jacket or pullover
- Medium-weight jacket
- All-weather boots (hiking style boots, over the ankle)

Medical Gear

Mimic the list I posted in the EDC Backpack. Be sure to have cutting shears, tourniquets, trauma dressings, blood-clotting agents, lots of gauze, lots of 4x4 bandages, minor wound treatment options, and antiseptic lotions or sprays.

Cash

Always have at least two hundred dollars cash in your Go-Bag in twenty-dollar bills. I know men who have gotten out of some extremely hazardous situations by throwing a couple of twenty-dollar bills at someone. This is especially true if you're traveling overseas. You never know when "greasing someone's palm" will be the easiest and fastest way to safety.

Light Source (Tactical Flashlight) and Extra Batteries

As mentioned earlier, everyone should have a good tactical flashlight and extra batteries. Another recommendation is having a "crank" flashlight—one that does not require batteries and you just repeatedly squeeze the handle or turn a crank to operate the flashlight.

Fire Source

I already described my homemade fire starter using petroleum jelly and cotton balls. You can also buy a good fire starter that comes in a toothpaste-style tube at your local outdoor store. Whatever you choose, always have a means to start a fire. Fire provides warmth and comfort. It also helps in signaling for rescue. Plus, you will need fire for boiling water and cooking. If you live in a cold region, fire may be your only answer against freezing temperatures.

Waterproof & Windproof Matches

In addition to a lighter, be sure to have matches on hand or a flint and stone to start your fire.

Signaling Mirror, Whistle, and Flares

In the event of an emergency, you will need a way to signal your location. A signal mirror can easily be seen for over twenty miles; a whistle can be heard over a mile away; and flares can attract attention both day and night.

Means to Purify Water

The American government has officially stated that a person requires at least one gallon of water per day for drinking and sanitation purposes. You should have a full two-liter water bottle in your Go-Bag. However, this water will only last for half a day or one day at most. After that, you need to find ways of purifying water—pack some water purification tablets (iodine tablets) or a compact purification tube. Such tubes are capable of filtering up to one thousand liters of water, and they remove 99.99 percent of bacteria. Or, choose a small filtered water pump that easily fits into your Go Bag.

Baby Wipes & Sanitation Supplies

Hygiene is very important during a crisis. If you fail to maintain it, you become prone to infections and contamination. Hence, your Go-Bag should definitely include a toilet paper roll, hand sanitizer, soap, and toothpaste/brush. Women should pack tampons or sanitary napkins too. Also include small bottles of body wash, shampoo, shaving cream, a razor, deodorant, sunscreen, body lotion, and a hair brush or comb.

Military Poncho & Poncho Liner

Go to your local Army Navy Store or order one on Amazon. This highly versatile and functional system is essential for every Go-Bag. It keeps you dry, warm, and concealed (camouflaged) and can also be used as a blanket, ground cover, temporary tent, or lean-to.

Candles & Chem-Lights

I have already described the benefits and many uses for Chem-Lights; however, having candles available is also a good idea. One burning candle inside your vehicle will keep the interior of your vehicle warm, without having to run the engine.

Duct Tape and Paracord

As detailed above.

Spare Batteries

If it uses batteries, you better have extra on hand!

Solar Charger for Cell Phone and Other Electronic Devices

These are cheap, lightweight, and do not require electricity or batteries.

Survival Knife

A good "Rambo-style" survival knife is a great tool with a multitude of uses.

Hunting Rifle and Spare Ammunition

I am a firm believer that everyone should know how to safely handle a firearm, particularly a hunting rifle. A semiautomatic bolt-action or lever-action rifle is inexpensive, easy-to-use, accurate both near and far, and great for hunting (you may need a food source) and could be the only solution needed to end violence perpetrated against you. Again, firearms will be discussed in a later chapter.

Items to Store in Your Vehicle

It should be obvious by now that I am a firm believer in the Boy Scout motto: "Be Prepared"; or in my world, the US Coast Guard motto: "Semper Paratus—Always Ready." I like to be prepared to deal with any crisis that may invade my daily routine. Having a few things on your person (everyday carry) is essential; however, having additional items in a backpack or laptop bag that is always within reach is another habit I encourage you to develop. Preparing for worst-case scenarios by packing a Go-Bag is yet another way to ensure your safety during a critical incident. The final "always ready" trick is to keep your vehicle geared up in the event you cannot get to your home and grab your Go-Bag.

Essentially, most everything in your Go-Bag should also be in your car's trunk. I also recommend you have the following:

A Spare Blanket
A blanket can help keep you warm, be used to build a shelter or as a ground cover, and be made into a stretcher if needed.

Bolt Cutters
If you need to cut through a chain link fence, cut off a padlock, or cut a cable, bolt cutters are essential. Think about it—if you're evacuating your home or city due to a major, life-threatening incident or catastrophe, you may need to cut a padlock or cut through a fence to get to safety.

Axe or Machete
A short-handled axe or machete is great for cutting small trees for firewood, clearing brush, and makes for a great weapon.

A Tool Box
Everyday tools such as screwdrivers, wrenches, pliers, socket wrenches, handsaws, and hammers, along with some screws, nails, bolts, and nuts can be a real lifesaver in an austere environment.

Extra Emergency Supplies
And if your vehicle has the room, don't be afraid to add extra water, medical supplies, food, and clothing.

Fuel
Final note on your vehicle: never let your gas tank get below half full. You never know when you're going to have to evacuate and you always want enough fuel to get you away from potential danger without having to refuel.

A lot of the items needed for your EDC backpack, Go-Bag, and in your vehicle can already be found in your home. The other items can be purchased over time. It is also important to know how to use each item you decide to pack.

Apps That Can Save Your Life

Today most people carry a cellphone. A cellphone is a great source of information as well as a communication tool. Countless lives have been saved with a cellphone's call for help.

Apple added a new emergency feature to their iPhone, which is designed to quickly and discreetly call emergency services. In the United States, "Emergency SOS" dials 911. Overseas, it works with local emergency response teams. Go into your "Settings" and scroll down till you see the "Emergency SOS" (This may be different for Android phones). Here you can set your phone to call your emergency contacts, provide your medical history, and decide how to initiate the SOS call. For my phone, I just push the right side button five times in rapid succession and my SOS call is initiated. It calls the local police with my location and notifies my emergency contacts.

These cellphone apps are truly beneficial when it comes to safety and security. There are apps that can take a photo of your would-be assailant, and then notify the assailant via the phone's speaker, that his photo has been taken, and the photo and the current location are being sent to the local police. Other apps track your location and send it a person of your choosing when you are traveling, on a run, or just out running errands. I don't want to endorse any single cellphone app, but there are several available that would be a great tool to help keep you and your loved ones safe.

Here are just a few:

- Family Locater: By LIFE360 basically works as a tracker. This location-sharing app keeps record of friends and family and places them on a map so everyone knows where they are at any given time. Of course, users within these circles can turn off their location-sharing feature at will. This app can be very helpful when traveling or roaming unfamiliar places. Family members can send automatic alerts to their circles when they arrive to their destination or they leave a certain place. They can also message each other and share to-do lists.

- Red Panic Button: In case of emergency press the Red Panic Button. This app can send an emergency message to any email or phone number with a press of a button. You can preset an emergency message and it will send your list of contacts an alert with your location. Red Panic Button is GPS based and will work on any network.

- SirenGPS: Did you know when you call 911, the dispatchers cannot track your exact location? They can only track you to the nearest cell phone tower. SirenGPS gives first responders access to your GPS location, and allows real-time, two-way communication between two people, even when cell phone service is down (which happens often during times of crisis, natural disasters, acts of terrorism, etc.).

- SafeTrek: Safe Trek is similar to SirenGPS, but simpler. This app consists of a single button you press and hold until you are in a safe location. If you let go of the button and do not enter a deactivation code within seconds, the app will contact local police. This app is great if you're constantly walking to a parking garage after work.

- Guardly Mobile: This app is more for organizations and work spaces, but still a good tool that can save lives. Guardly Mobile can be used by security operators and dispatchers to send emergency and operational alerts to staff and members in a crisis. For example, if there were an active shooter at a mall, a security operator can send a critical alert to all mall employees so that they are aware. Emergency alerts can also be used for fires, theft, and even severe weather forecasts.

Gun or No Gun?

Do I get a concealed handgun license or do I not?

I am asked this question more than any other question in my training courses. My response is always the same. I ask them, "Do you have life insurance? Do you wear a seatbelt when you drive? Do you lock your doors at night? Do you have health insurance, car insurance? Do you have smoke detectors in your home or a fire extinguisher in your kitchen? Does your car have an airbag?" Undoubtedly, most of the replies I get to all these questions are "yes".

Then I ask them, "So you have all these plans and take all these precautions to protect yourself in case bad things happen, right? What is your plan if really, really bad things happen like a carjacking, home invasion, or armed robbery?"

I usually hear the deafening sound of silence. They have no response because they know they are living in a state of denial that "it will never happen to me." Most people do have insurance and drive with a seatbelt and have smoke detectors in their home, but they don't have a weapon available to them should they ever need it. Are the chances of having a house fire any greater than a home invasion? Most people are prepared for the fire, but not for the night of violence.

I think every American citizen of sound mind and body should have a weapon in their home and in their vehicle. I believe that if this were the case, the violent crime rate in America would plummet due to the violent offenders being afraid of an armed victim. Of course there would need to be strict regulations about the safe storage of the weapons, and we would have to do a much better job educating our children on weapon safety, but those are hurdles easily overcome.

There is an old saying in the Special Operations community that says, "It is better to have it and not need it than need it and not have it." I feel this is exactly the reasoning and rationale for everyone to have (and know how to use) a handgun. The truth is if you need a handgun, and don't have one, you are in a world of trouble!

If you do decide to arm yourself, it is your responsibility to be proficient with that weapon—period. No exceptions. No excuses. You will need to follow a strict training regimen to safely and effectively carry a concealed handgun. No matter what your state's minimum requirements are for you to legally carry a weapon, they will NOT meet my standards. My standards are much higher. I truly believe if you carry a weapon and you are not firing at least two thousand rounds a year (five hundred rounds a quarter), plus taking a tactical handgun training course at least twice a year, then you are not taking the responsibility of owning a handgun seriously.

Shooting is a perishable and diminishing skill. If you don't use it, you lose it. I should know, I shot thousands of rounds a week while a member of the FBI's Hostage Rescue Team, and I was extremely good at my job—that is, surgical shooting. Now that I've retired from the FBI, I do not shoot even a thousand rounds a month, and I know I am not the shooter I used to be. No one can master and maintain a skill without practice, commitment, and dedication. This is also true of shooting.

The decision to carry a firearm is not something to be taken lightly. It is a huge commitment and one that will have dire consequences if not taken seriously. To have your weapon taken from you, especially if you are untrained or unskilled in the art of using a weapon, creates a real threat, not only to you, but to those around you.

Conclusion

There isn't a one-size-fits-all in deciding your daily essentials. What you carry also depends on where you live (state laws for gun and knife carry vary greatly) and how much you're willing to train. Again, although I carry a handgun with me at all times, I DO NOT recommend you carry one unless you are licensed and trained to carry a weapon.

Remember, "Survival is not a skill set; it's a mindset." Start thinking about what you want to have available at any given moment, under any circumstance.

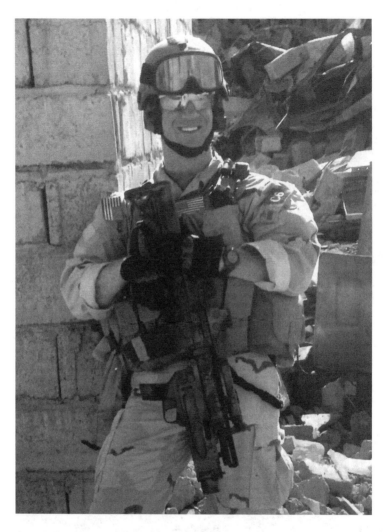

Figure 2 Greg Shaffer (HRT) in Falluja, Iraq; circa 2003

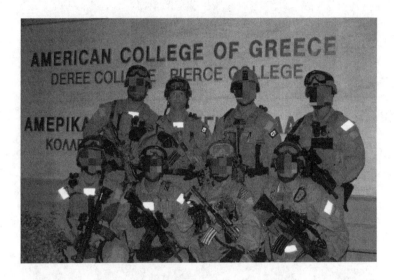

Figure 3 Greg Shaffer and FBI HRT during the 2004 Summer Olympic Games; Athens, Greece

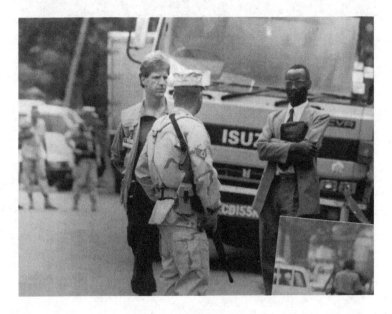

Figure 4 Greg Shaffer in Nairobi, Kenya following the 1998 U.S. Embassy bombing

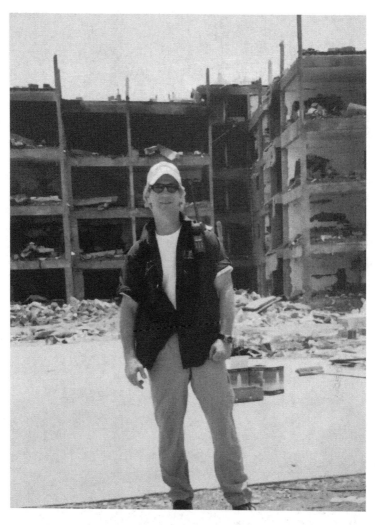

Figure 5 Greg Shaffer in Saudi Arabia for the US/UK Housing Complex Bombings, 2003

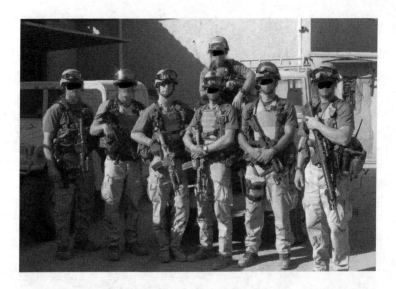

Figure 6 Greg Shaffer and HRT in Iraq, circa 2003

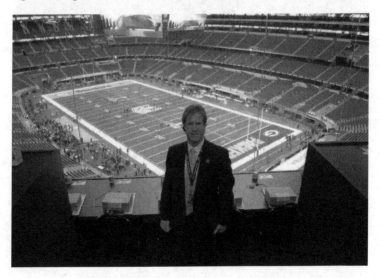

Figure 7 Greg Shaffer, FBI Supervisor for the 2011 NFL Super Bowl

Part 2

HOW TO "STAY SAFE"

Chapter 4
TRAVEL SECURITY

There is a greater travel risk now than in the past, but by taking a few precautions you and your family can safely enjoy this great big, beautiful world. Statistically, you are far more likely to become a victim of crime or be involved in a vehicle accident than to be a victim of terrorism. Still, the threat of terrorism, whether it is Islamic radicalism or narco-terrorism from the drug cartels, is real and cannot be ignored and Americans will be targeted.

Again, your greatest threat while traveling is from car accidents and petty crimes such as pickpocketing and purse snatching. The most common injury sustained overseas is not from terrorism or kidnapping, but from vehicle accidents. Every time you cross the street, get into a cab, rent a moped, or drive a car in a foreign country, your risk of injury increases dramatically. Some data suggests over 90 percent of injuries for American tourist overseas is related to a moving vehicle accident. When you get into a taxi, Uber car, or limousine, you are putting your life into someone else's hands. Your situational awareness and a heightened sense of your environment are critical during this time. By now you should have learned that when you get into a taxi in a foreign country, you should have your tactical pen in hand and have discussed with your travel companion what actions to take during certain situations.

Another common incident that affects over fifteen million travelers per year is natural disasters, mostly earthquakes. Be sure to have your important documents, as discussed in chapter 3, photographed and downloaded onto your phone and in the cloud, and keep a paper copy on your person or locked in the front desk safe of your hotel. A natural disaster could interrupt cellphone service for days, if not weeks. However, don't let the fear of earthquakes, terrorism, or kidnapping prevent you from enjoying world travel. You have a much greater risk of injury while crossing the street—and that's avoidable with good situational awareness!

Collect Pre-Travel Intelligence

Before you decide to travel, be sure to spend some time doing your "pre-travel intelligence collection," also known as "ground truth." That is, determine whether or not it is safe for you to travel to that destination. A comprehensive "threat analysis" should be done prior to your departure. Do not let the term "threat analysis" intimidate you.

Gathering information and intelligence off the internet makes this process fairly easy and painless. If you are traveling overseas, consider the following US Department of State websites before departing:

- US Department of State Smart Traveler Enrollment Program (https://step.state.gov/step/): The Smart Traveler Enrollment Program (STEP) is a free service to allow US citizens traveling abroad to enroll their trip with the US Department of State. This enrollment will allow you to receive information from the embassy about safety conditions in your destination country and help you make informed decisions about your travel plans.

- For a list of the nearest US Embassy or Consulate for each destination, go to: http://www.usembassy.gov/.
- A copy of your destination's "911 emergency equivalent" phone numbers for police, fire, and ambulance support can be found at: http://travel.state.gov/content/dam/students-abroad/pdfs/911_ABROAD.pdf.

Another effective way to learn about a location you want to visit is to ask friends. Get as much information as you can from people who live there or have been there recently. Go online and read the local newspapers from the city you are about to visit. In addition, when you are en route, strike up a conversation with the passengers next to you on the flight. They can offer you valuable insights and provide recommendations for places to see, restaurants to visit, and areas you want to avoid.

Your intelligence collection should include the following:

- What is the location of the nearest hospital and police station to your hotel?
- Where is the US Embassy or Consulate?
- What type of public transportation is best to use?
- Will you have cell phone coverage to implement your "communications plan" (to be discussed shortly) if needed?
- How far is the airport from your hotel? Knowing this and tracking your taxi ride on Google Maps is a good way to ensure you are taking the most direct, cheapest, and secure route. We will discuss later in this chapter about how getting into a taxi in a foreign country can be one of the most dangerous aspects of travel.

As I mentioned in the previous chapter, you will want to have important documents such as your passport, credit cards, medical information, prescriptions, driver's license, insurance, and contact information for family and friends uploaded in the cloud and on your cell phone for easy access. I don't know about you, but I can't recite the phone number of anyone other than my wife from memory. Our smartphones have allowed us to become lazy in our memorizing phone numbers. I remember as a teenager I could recite the telephone numbers for over twenty of my friends. Not now! Be sure those important phone numbers are written down and available in the event your phone is lost or stolen.

It is important to obtain as much information on the country you are about to visit prior to departure. I know this sounds elementary and obvious, but you would be surprised how many travelers get in trouble at Customs and Immigration because they are carrying something illicit for that country, which could have been easily identified had they conducted pre-travel intelligence collection. Information is knowledge and knowledge is power.

Finally, don't forget your vaccinations! You may be required to have certain vaccinations prior to entry. For a complete list of what is needed prior to travel and recommended by the Center for Disease Control (CDC), go to: http://wwwnc.cdc.gov/travel/destinations/list.

In determining the "Ground Truth" (gaining knowledge, information, and intelligence on the location you are visiting) consider these points:

- Terrorist attacks can be predicted. Previous terrorist attack sites should be avoided as well as previous attack anniversary dates. Know if any previous attacks have occurred, at which locations and on what dates—avoid as necessary.

- Terrorists often target transportation hubs. Other targets include government buildings (US Embassies), Western hotel chains, high-profile events, nightclubs, and places frequented by Westerners. Know where these areas are and try to avoid them.

- Know that "industrial espionage" exists everywhere, especially in China, Russia, India, France, and Israel. Do not travel with sensitive, proprietary information you do not want compromised.

- Assume you are being monitored. Many countries will monitor all of your communications and movements. Foreign governments may also monitor your internet, usage, cell phone calls, and public places commonly used by tourists.

- Medical care and food and water quality are frequently substandard in developing countries. When in doubt, only drink bottled water and refrain from iced drinks. Avoid fruits and vegetables that may have been rinsed with tap water.

- Avoid contact with birds, dogs, insects, or wildlife. They may carry many viruses and diseases you want to avoid. If possible, stay away from all animals while on foreign soil.

- Know what is legal and what is illegal prior to entering the Customs area. Prohibited items: Most countries have restrictions on items as satellite phones, bullet-resistant clothing, weapons, restraints, and some medical items (including medications).

- Generally, civil unrest occurs in the same locations in a given city. The government may allow people to only protest in designated areas. Avoid these areas.

- Transportation unions around the world often go on strike. Most of these are announced prior to their execution. Know your ground truth.
- Tourism equals crime. Tourists are more likely to be a target of petty crime than anyone else. There will be petty crime wherever there are tourists.
- Female travel safety can be especially concerning, depending on your location. Know the culture and customs of the country you are visiting before you leave home.
- Every country has some corrupt law enforcement officers, some more than others.
- Nothing you leave in the hotel room is safe: your laptop, data on the laptop, USB drives, phones, wallets, jewelry—nothing.

Use common sense security practices and always practice situational awareness.

Load Your Apps

As I said earlier, using your cellphone's capabilities is a great way to help you in maintaining good situational awareness and critical incident response. There are apps that help you stay informed during a crisis, which may be developing in the country or area you are visiting. These apps can provide a "country profile" with information on the culture, language, and interesting things to do and see. They can also alert you to any dangerous weather, disease outbreaks, infrastructure outages, or civil unrest. Many have a panic button that communicates your location while summoning assistance. These apps do not replace travel insurance, which covers the cost of a medical emergency or evacuation, but they do provide a range of services designed to keep travelers safe.

Another useful app is a currency converter. I find it difficult to mentally convert local currency into US dollars, especially when I am traveling to several countries. A simple currency converter app shows you how much things cost in US dollars, and can help you avoid spending too much.

Google Translate and Google Maps are also fantastic apps to have at your fingertips. Being able to translate street signs or a restaurant menu can save you a lot of frustration. Using Google Maps is a good way to track where you are going, even if you are in a cab, on the subway, or walking the streets. Just be sure to maintain your situational awareness and do not get distracted by your mobile device.

Be sure to turn on all the security measures of your cell phone prior to travel. Activate the remote locate and lock features, which are standard on most smartphones, so that you can disable your device if it is lost or stolen. You will want a secure password that opens your phone and uses uppercase, lowercase, numbers, and special characters. You want to enable the Find My Phone app, and have the phone lock itself if more than seven attempts are made with an incorrect password. Do not use a pattern lock on your device. Most of those can be broken in five attempts or less. Finally, be sure to install or update the latest anti-malware program on all the devices you are taking with you.

Develop a Communications Plan

Imagine this: Your spouse goes missing after a catastrophic earthquake. A bus carrying students is involved in a fatal accident in an area in which you know you child is traveling. Cell-phone coverage has gone down or is nonexistent. A terrorist attack closes a major international airport where your parents are due to land. Each of these realistic scenarios can quickly turn an exciting vacation, study abroad program, or business trip into a personal or organizational crisis.

When the moment of crisis has arrived,

the time for planning has passed.

Always have a plan.

The importance of a "communications plan" established prior to travel has always been a good idea, but even more so in today's world with the many recent terrorist attacks, natural disasters, and civil unrest. Having a "comms plan" (communications plan) is a must-have item on your checklist prior to travel.

The first and most important component of your comms plan is to ensure your emergency contact has your travel itinerary, which includes flight information, hotels, in-country points of contact, and a photocopy of your passport and driver's license.

I have already discussed how many of us no longer have important telephone numbers memorized. They are maintained in our cellphones, and if we ever lost our phones or had them stolen, most of us would be at a loss to remember an emergency contact number. So, I remind you, keep a written list of your contact names, addresses, and phone numbers on your person as well as in your phone when traveling. Keep the same list uploaded into the cloud for access via the internet. Your contact list should also have the number for the US Embassy in every country you are visiting. Be sure everyone traveling with you has a copy of your communication plan and your contacts in case you get separated.

Establish a phone tree, so if you are only able to contact one person, that person knows to call the others on your list to advise them of your situation or needs.

Establish a social media platform on which to communicate your status. It could be on a private Facebook page or a Twitter account. You may not always have access to the internet, but if you do, a simple note to your family on social media will alleviate a lot of their concerns about your safety.

Set up regular "check-in" times. That is, establish a communication plan where you phone your emergency contact every night at 8:00 p.m. local time, or at noon, on even-numbered days of the month. If you miss two consecutive call-ins, your emergency contact should start initiating the phone tree to see if anyone else has heard from you. If not, emergency procedures to locate you may be considered.

A text message may get through on your cellphone when a phone call may not, and text messages require less bandwidth than a phone call. Also, text messages automatically save themselves and will go out (send) when bandwidth becomes available.

Another part of your comms plan is to store at least one emergency contact under the name "In Case of Emergency" or "ICE" in your mobile phone. This will help someone identify your emergency contact if you are unable to do so because of injury or illness. Be sure to let your emergency contact know of any medical issues or other requirements you may have.

Remember your "duress word" and be sure your emergency contact knows what it is and what to do if you use that word in a text or phone call.

During your trip, both you and your emergency contact (and you may want to have more than one) should routinely monitor local news outlets as well as the websites detailed above. Special attention should be given to signs of civil unrest, inclement weather, terrorist attacks in the region, and major natural or man-made disasters. Be sure you can retrieve your emails while traveling, as they can be a great source of information on pending issues relating to security. Avoid traveling with your laptop in a laptop bag. Instead, use a common, nondescript bag that won't attract the attention of a thief. Be careful of free Wi-Fi in public places, as they are rarely secure. Do all your computer related work in the privacy of your hotel room or at the local branch of your firm. And never leave your computer in your hotel room when it is unoccupied. Not only is it inviting theft, but the data on it could be easily stolen and result in identity theft or proprietary information being released. Finally, either carry your computer everywhere you go, or have the concierge put it in the hotel safe. Remember, room safes are not safe at all!

Do not hesitate to reschedule your trip, or cut your trip short if a significant health or safety concern arises.

Stay Safe as an Airline Passenger

Flying is still the safest way to travel. Experts say the chance of being killed in a major airline crash is one in five million. Those are pretty good odds! Despite that, incidents do happen and you need to be prepared to take the appropriate action. Although it is rare that passengers will have to evacuate a commercial airliner, when it is necessary, you must do so as quickly and as efficiently as possible.

"Dress for success"—by this I mean dress so that you can successfully survive an airline catastrophe. Do not wear sandals; wear comfortable shoes that can be tied tight and have good traction in the event of an emergency. Men should wear a pair of good sturdy slacks, such as blue jeans, dungarees, or cargo pants. Women should not wear long, loose clothing that can get snagged or hung up in the event of an emergency evacuation. Clothing can be stylish and practical.

Before an airline receives Federal Aviation Administration (FAA) certification, they must show that passengers are able to exit the aircraft quickly and safely in compliance with regulations. Over the years, the FAA has upgraded cabin safety requirements to ensure that more passengers will survive an aviation accident. All US commercial airplanes have numerous FAA-required safety features: floor path emergency lighting, fire-resistant seat cushions, low heat and smoke release cabin materials, and improved cabin insulation. Each of these improvements give passengers and crew more time to make a speedy evacuation.

Federal regulations specify that the manufacturer of an airplane with more than forty-four passenger seats must be able to evacuate a full airplane, under emergency conditions, within ninety seconds. Ninety seconds?

I took this photograph on a recent domestic flight while I was writing this chapter. In this photo you can see the over-wing emergency exits. They are five rows away. There are six people per row, five rows in front and five rows in back of the wing exits, with only one aisle to get to the exit. That equates to sixty people moving to the aisle to get off the plane, and out of those four little window exits. My seat was five rows from the over-wing emergency exits and I thought to myself, "There is no way I would be able to get out of this aircraft in less than ninety seconds, and I am only five rows from the door." The panic and chaos that would ensue, and the mass of bodies attempting to get off the plane would clog the over-wing doors almost instantly. In my opinion, the way the commercial airline industry has jammed more and more seats into an aircraft makes it virtually impossible for a ninety-second evacuation.

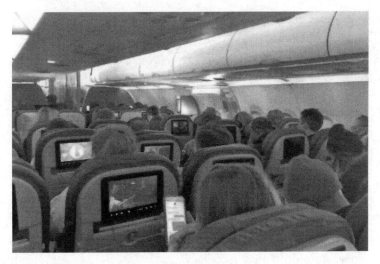

Figure 8 Note the location of the Over-Wing Exits

Over the years the airlines have continually reduced the amount of leg room in order to get more paying customers on board. Have they done this at the expense of safety? I am not a certified FAA Safety Evaluator, but I do know human nature and I know the size of those over-wing doors and I do not believe an aircraft of this size could be evacuated in one-and-a-half minutes.

The good news is that flying is an incredibly safe way to travel so your chances of being in an emergency situation on board a commercial airliner are very slim. On the other hand, always have a plan! Listen to the emergency evacuation instructions prior to takeoff. Pull out the safety card in the seat back in front of you and study the floor plan of the plane, taking note of the locations of two exits, and know how to operate (open) the doors. No matter how often you fly, always read the safety card prior to take-off because every aircraft is different and not all airplane doors open the same way.

It has been shown that most passengers in an aircraft accident do not die from a violent crash. Most deaths are a result of smoke inhalation. Therefore, it is critical to get out of the plane as quickly as you can. When making airline reservations, choose your seat closest to an emergency exit and learn how to open that emergency door. Know how to open it even if the cabin is filled with dense, black smoke! "To Move is to Live; to Freeze is to Die."

Under stress, you have only three responses—Freeze, Fight, or Flight. You do not want to get stuck in a burning, smoke-filled plane behind someone who is frozen in fear. Sit near an exit.

Stay Safe Traveling in Vehicles

The biggest risk to any traveler in a foreign country is vehicular accidents, whether it is from being struck by a vehicle while crossing the street, getting ambushed in the back of a taxi, or being involved in a motor vehicle accident. Most injuries to travelers in a foreign country involve a motor vehicle—I know this firsthand!

In 2006 I learned a hard lesson on how important situational awareness is to your health and well-being. I was invited to speak at a Pan-Pacific Counter Terrorism conference in Sydney, Australia. I flew from Washington, DC, to Sydney on an overnight flight. I arrived early in the morning Australian time. I didn't want to sleep when I arrived because I wanted to get acclimated to the time zone, so I pushed through the morning, went for a nice long run along the Sydney waterfront during lunch, and then went out for an early dinner around 5:30 p.m. I was tired and jet-lagged. While I was walking back to my hotel after leaving the restaurant, I was almost killed by a speeding taxi. As I started to cross the street, I looked left (forgetting that in Australia, I needed to look right) and stepped into the road. I forgot that the Aussies drive on the "wrong side of the road." I was hit by a taxi traveling at 40 mph and thrown into the air. I barely cheated death, but I did suffer horribly. I was not able to attend the next day's conference, and I had to have emergency surgery in a Sydney hospital.

My Aussie taxi experience was a direct result of me letting my guard down. I was operating in "Condition White," on autopilot, unaware of my surroundings. It is easy to get complacent and drop your guard. I was certainly operating on autopilot that evening; and it nearly cost me my life.

On a side note to that story, I want to publically thank the Director of the Australian Federal Police for sending me a bottle of fine scotch to assist in my recovery after my surgery. It certainly helped ease the pain. Cheers, mate!

Taxis

There are countless stories of kidnappings, abductions, and violent crime taking place in the back of a foreign taxi. Even today it is not safe to get into a cab in Rio de Janiero. My dear friend Martha, who travels the world over 250 days a year on business, was violently assaulted and robbed in the back of a taxi in South America. While sitting in the back of the taxi at a stoplight, her assailant opened the rear door and got in. He took her purse and jewelry but not before hitting her several times in the face and chest. Although the cab driver claimed complete innocence when questioned by the police, I'm sure he got his "cut" from the robber later that night. Her only mistake was not having a plan before she got in the taxi. Could she have locked the rear doors? Could she have had her tactical pen in hand? Could she have hired a vetted driver, one provided by the hotel, and not hailed a public taxi?

Keep in mind, most robberies, abductions, and violent crime occurs in or near a vehicle. It is, therefore essential that you maintain your situational awareness when selecting a taxi, getting into a taxi, or traveling in a taxi. Always have a plan and, in some cases, have your tactical pen in hand when getting into a cab.

Always find out which cab companies are legitimate when you are traveling. Most cities have safe, clean, licensed, professional taxis sources; but there's always the chance of the fly-by-night, "put a sign on the door and call yourself a taxi" nonprofessionals or even crooks looking for a fare. Be sure you know the "ground truth."

The risks of kidnapping, robbery, and sexual assault are significantly reduced if you do not have to hail taxis. However, sometimes taxis are the only option.

- *First rule when using a taxi*: Never let anyone direct you to the taxi. You choose the taxi cab and if possible, never choose the taxi that is first in the queue.
- *Second rule when using a taxi:* Never get into an unmarked taxi. Always make sure the taxi is well marked, uses a meter, and has the license of the driver prominently displayed. Be sure to ask your hotel's concierge to recommend a cab company and have their phone number readily available. Calling for a cab is always better than hailing one off the street corner, especially in foreign countries.

Another option I highly recommend is to find a licensed, insured, and reputable driving service. It is not always easy to find a trusted and vetted private driver, but if you know someone in-country who can recommend a driving service, and it is within your budget, please use them. It is one of the single best ways to stay safe while in a foreign country. A well-trusted, professional livery driver will prevent you from wandering into areas that are not safe; they will quickly and safely get you from point A to point B; they can keep your hands free by locking your laptops or bags in the trunk of the vehicle; and they prevent you from being robbed by unscrupulous cab drivers and car-jackers.

Rental Cars

If you decide to rent a vehicle, be sure you hide your maps and guidebooks when you park your car, get fuel, or stop for a bite to eat. Put them in the glove box or under a coat in the back seat. The same goes for English-language newspapers, directions, or reading material. You want your vehicle, as well as yourself, to blend in with the local environment.

While in your rental vehicle, avoid parking garages, which are known to be popular haunts for criminals, especially overseas. Be sure to park your car in a well-lit area, or use a valet service when available.

The final word on renting a vehicle overseas: always, always, always get the liability insurance! Regardless of your private auto insurance, regardless of your firm's policy, regardless of how safe a driver you think you are—pay the additional small fee and get the insurance. There are countless numbers of cases where vacations have been ruined due to a rental car accident. Taking the pre-offered liability insurance would have saved them a lot of headaches and a lot of money.

Blend In—Don't Stick Out

If you're traveling overseas—leave the University of Florida tee shirt at home. Bringing attention to yourself as a "tourist" is not what you want to do in a foreign country. This includes sweatshirts, baseball hats, and leggings that scream "Hey, I'm an American tourist!" Don't make yourself an easy target; blend into the environment as much as you can. The best and easiest way to blend (remember good guys and bad guys look for the anomalies while establishing a baseline for their environment) is to alter your appearance; therefore, dress, eat, and play like the locals. Learn a few phrases in the language before you depart. A simple "thank you," "good day," and "please" in the native tongue goes a long way in being welcomed by the local populous. Plus, you don't stick out as the obnoxious tourist. Do what you can to blend into the environment and leave the Hawaiian shirt at home.

Another way to blend in is to use the local currency. Be sure to convert your US dollars to local currency before you leave the airport. You may not be able to pay for the taxi or bus or subway with US dollars. You will want to have some local currency for tips when you check in at your hotel as well. Just be sure not to flash a lot of money around at the currency counter; you never know who may be watching.

Know Where to Stay

I am often asked, "Isn't it more dangerous to stay in an American hotel overseas? Aren't they targeted more by terrorists?" The answer is yes, in some countries that may be true. And if it is true, maybe you should reconsider traveling to that country. However, in reality, the greatest risk you will face while traveling overseas is petty crime, car accidents, and food poisoning, and these threats tend to be less at US hotel chains. Many US hotel chains conduct rigorous background checks on their employees, which cut down on burglary, assaults, and petty crimes. They also have stricter sanitary requirements, so you are less likely to suffer from food contamination. Nothing ruins a successful business trip or fun-filled vacation worse than food poisoning.

Another consideration for staying in a US-based hotel is many have on-site or on-call physicians who speak English, and can attend to you in a medical emergency.

When you are checking in or making the reservation, ask for a room on the third to sixth floor. The rooms located on the first and second floors tend to be targeted by burglars due to the easy escape from these floors. The third through sixth floor rooms are less inviting to thieves yet still allow access for most fire engine ladder trucks to reach you. Hotel fires are not as uncommon as you may think. The knowledge that a fireman can reach you in a time of crisis is a comforting thought.

Avoid rooms near the stairwells. These are often targeted by thieves due to the ease of a quick getaway. If possible, avoid rooms with sliding doors. Sliding doors can give you a nice view, but they are also an invitation for criminals, kidnappers, and terrorists. If you have no option and your room has a sliding door, use a dresser drawer for added security. Remove the empty drawer, lay it along the track of the sliding door, and push it squarely into the corner of the doorframe.

Once you get to your room, before you unpack your belongings, walk the hallway to the nearest emergency exit—probably a stairwell. Be sure you know the route so that you can find the exit even if you are on your knees and the hallway is filled with dense black smoke. In the event of a hotel fire, soak all the towels in water and put them over your shoulders and head, with a wet cloth over your nose and mouth, before attempting to exit your room.

If the fire is in the hallway and you cannot escape your room, put wet towels and blankets on the floor against the bottom of the door. Use a wet towel and swing it around the room to catch smoke particles. Watch for emergency personnel and try to get their attention. Once the emergency teams have arrived, use your tactical pen to break the window—remember to puncture the window in a corner, not in the middle. Break the window only if you are having trouble breathing. An open window can create a natural draft that could suck more smoke into your room. If you do not have a tactical pen, use a lamp or break the leg off the desk or a chair. Signal the firefighters from your window by waving a sheet or use a piece of mirror broken off the bathroom mirror or vanity. If part of your travel EDC (everyday carry) is a whistle and a flashlight, use those to signal for help.

An often overlooked benefit of staying in hotels is to use the concierge desk. Use them as your personal command post. The concierge is knowledgeable and can recommend places to eat, what to see, where to go, and can advise you regarding areas of the city you should avoid. If you are going to be in town for an extended stay, they can help you access the hotel driver service, or recommend a livery service for you to hire. Have the concierge keep your valuables, such as your laptop, contact list, and credit cards (in a sealed envelope) in the hotel safe. Remember, you should be carrying only one form of identification and one or two credit cards in your wallet in the event it is misplaced or stolen.

Be sure to keep the business card of your hotel in your front pocket when you leave for the day. It won't be stolen if your wallet is taken; you can show the card to a taxi driver and know he's going to take you to the right hotel; and you now have an emergency contact number for your new best friend—the hotel's concierge.

Travel with Weapons—Improvised Weapons!

It is very easy to travel with weapons if you use a little ingenuity. I recommend to all my clients to never travel without having a few weapons on hand. These improvised weapons can be taken on aircraft and are easily explained to any Customs Officer anywhere in the world.

Improvised weapons include the following:

Tactical/Unbreakable Umbrella

The most robust umbrella you will ever own. Not only will it protect you from the elements, it will also protect you in case of an emergency. For less than $100.00 you can purchase an outstanding personal defense weapon that can be carried with you worldwide. I recommend the umbrella with the rounded, ball-shaped handle, not the cane-style or curved handle.

Tactical Pen

As previously discussed, these pens—made from titanium—are indispensable and should be a part of your Every Day Carry (EDC). You can purchase most tactical pens for around $25.00.

Large Carabiner

I clip a carabiner on the outside of my backpack and hang a ball cap off of it. It looks harmless; however, placing the carabiner across your fist makes for a good "brass knuckle"-type striking device.

Shemagh/Scarf and a Large Padlock

Slip the scarf or *shemagh* (also known as a keffiyeh) through the padlock, halfway down the length of the scarf. Tie the two ends together and start swinging. Note: When going through a security checkpoint, be sure the padlock and the scarf and not connected.

Once in country, visit a local hardware store and buy a large Phillips-head screwdriver; an ice pick, or an eight-inch length of one-inch diameter lead pipe.

Learn to Be Street Smart

Vacations are a time to relax. Do not let the desire (or need) for rest and relaxation diminish your situational awareness. Do not let down your guard. Stay alert, "Live in the Yellow," so that you can enjoy a safe, secure, relaxing vacation or a successful business trip. Use common sense and a little "street savvy" to stay safe. I discussed earlier about not letting anyone direct you to a specific taxi. Here are a few other ways to be "street smart":

- Do not change your American dollars into local currency from the guy on the street corner! If he does not rob you (which is often the case), then the police may arrest you— it is illegal in most countries to exchange money on the black market.
- Always have enough local coins in your pocket to make a phone call. You never know when you are going to lose your phone or have it stolen. It is always nice to have enough coins to call your hotel and ask them to send a taxi or driver for you.
- Stay away from public disturbances or civil unrest. I know it sounds obvious, but don't let a large, boisterous crowd entice you to see what is going on. A loud, public disturbance is the kind of trouble you want to avoid and could be a ruse used by a gang of pickpockets and purse snatchers.
- As I previously mentioned, keep the fact that you are a tourist to a minimum. That includes not putting your nation's flag on your backpack or wearing a Stars and Stripes baseball cap.
- Beware of unsolicited advice, directions, street beggars, or anyone wanting to practice their English. In these situations, be sure to have control of your purse and wallet.
- Always prepare to travel with this thought: If you don't want it stolen, don't take it with you. This includes expensive jewelry, wedding rings, heirlooms, watches, and purses.

Pickpockets come in all shapes and sizes. Some of the best pickpockets I have seen are ten-to-twelve-year-old kids who work in teams and are as smooth as silk when stealing your wallet. Therefore, do not carry all your cash and all your credit cards in one place. Put some in your wallet, some in your front pocket, and maybe leave some in a sealed envelope in the hotel safe.

A good pre-travel checklist prior to departing overseas is to have your "Four Cs" covered: Credentials, Cash, Communications, and Contacts.

- Your credentials include your passport, driver's license, proof of insurance, and business cards. You also want to have a photo of each of these uploaded into the cloud and on your cell phone.
- Cash is king, especially during a crisis or critical situation. Always have at least two hundred dollars in twenty-dollar bills in a money belt, in your shoe, or in your front pocket. As I mentioned before, greasing someone's palm can often be the safest, most expedient way to get out of a jam. Keep in mind, this money is only for emergency situations.
- You need to be able to communicate during your travels, so be sure you have extra cell phone batteries, wall adapters, converters, and other equipment needed to keep your phone charged and functional. Be sure all the necessary apps are loaded and the most current malware is loaded onto your device.
- Keep a contact list on your phone, in your wallet, at the front desk of your hotel, and uploaded into the cloud. You should have access to your emergency contact list no matter the circumstance. If you are ever in a position where you need your contact list, chances are you are REALLY going to need it! This list should contain both contact telephone numbers and emails.

Please do not let this chapter scare you into never leaving the house! There is a great big, beautiful world out there with incredible sights, amazing people, and wonderful foods—all to be explored. With a little research and prior planning, you can travel the world safely and return with tales of adventure.

Chapter 5
HOME & VEHICLE SECURITY

Did you know that a home burglary occurs every fourteen seconds in the United States? That is more than two million burglaries each year, and one-third of these burglars enter the home through an unlocked door or window (FBI 2015). Children go in and out of the house all day long, leaving the doors open. So do adults who pop next door for a quick visit or take the dog for a walk. It always surprises me to learn how many families routinely leave their doors unlocked, especially when they are in the house. Always, always, always keep your doors locked—particularly when you are in the home! Items such as televisions, computers, and jewelry can be replaced with an insurance claim; your life is not replaceable. Please keep your doors locked when you are in your home. It's unfortunate we must do this, but it's the reality of the world in which we live.

Home Security Tricks
There are several obvious ways to burglar-proof your home: have your neighbor pick up your mail and newspapers everyday while you're away; purchase electronic timers that turn your lights on and off at specific hours; or go wireless and set up your home so you can turn on lights, control the thermostat, and use voice

commands through an exterior speaker, all from your smartphone. However, although these nuggets are extremely beneficial, they are widely known and have become more common sense than "tricks of the trade."

It is a widely publicized fact that 85 percent of burglars case the homes they intend to rob (FBI 2015). They do a reconnaissance of the neighborhood prior to their crime, in order to identify which homes will be targeted, so make your home unattractive to burglars. Take a walk through your neighborhood in the evening with the mindset of a criminal. During the walk, think like a thief and ask yourself, "Which houses look empty? Which homes have their front doorways hidden due to poorly trimmed landscaping? Which houses have mail or newspapers stuffed in their mailboxes? Who leaves their garage doors open?" Trust me; you'll be able to identify which homes are more susceptible to burglaries and which are not. Take note of what caught your attention and ensure you prep your home accordingly. Most burglars are criminals of opportunity. They are always looking for the easy score. Make them choose another softer, easier target.

Sociologists have interviewed convicted burglars and found three common factors they use to decide which home to burglarize: time, noise, and visibility. Professional burglars want to get in and out of your home as quickly as possible. So, the more difficult it is to pick your lock, the longer it takes the burglar to break in. The longer it takes, the better it is for you.

Besides the time factor, thieves also do not want to be noticed. They don't want anything to draw attention to their actions. A dog barking, motion alarms, or a home security system, all create noise. Burglars will often by-pass a home with a barking dog for a quieter environment.

Visibility is also an important factor thieves consider when deciding who to rob. Homes that are poorly lit, don't have motion sensor lighting, or have large shrubs and bushes near the doors and windows all create ideal opportunities for the burglar.

Time, noise, visibility—the more you can increase these factors, the less likely your home will be targeted for burglary.

Lights, Locks & Doors

Keeping your home well-lit from the outside and installing good locks will go a long way in keeping your home safe from burglars. The typical locks you buy at Home Depot or Lowe's are substandard and easily picked by the most novice lock picker—usually in less than thirty seconds. Although a good lock may cost you a little extra, it is well worth it for the peace of mind you get knowing it takes time to defeat. The BiLock, Mul-T-Lock, or Medeco are just a few of the better locks on the market that can frustrate even an experienced locksmith. Do your own research regarding which lock to purchase. And if you find you have a Kwikset or Schlage front and rear door lock, you may want to replace them with a sturdier, more durable lock.

Walk around the perimeter of your own property at night, and look for areas where thieves may hide. Once those areas are identified, place motion detector lighting in those places. Motion detector lighting is easy to install and is very effective in thwarting thieves.

If you have doors with glass panes, or sliding glass doors, be sure to put security film on the windows. This film is clear, tear-resistant, virtually nondetectable and keeps the glass together if a thief is trying to break the glass. Also, use double-cylinder locks on doors with windows. These locks require a key on both the inside and outside of the door. Just be sure not to leave the key in the lock where the thief can reach inside and turn the key to open your door. However, keep in mind that in a fire or other crisis which may require a hasty evacuation, the cylinder lock will require a key to get out.

French doors look nice, but are inherently unsafe and very easy to kick open because of their split door design. In addition, French doors are mostly glass, which is easily overcome by seasoned burglars. The same goes for sliding glass doors; they are great for letting in light and for the views, but they can be easily lifted off their tracks by even inexperienced thieves. If you have sliding glass doors, be sure to buy an after-market locking device to secure the door.

Always keep your garage door shut unless you are outside the house where you can view it at all times. There was a horrific home invasion in Indiana where four robbers entered the home through an open garage door. They terrorized the family, raped and assaulted both the wife and daughter, and killed the husband.

Keep your garage door closed, as well as the access door into your home from the garage. This is crucial. When you are going to be away from home for any extended time, I recommend you disengage the automatic garage door opener and use the attached garage door lock or a padlock to secure it.

Package Deliveries

There are far too many stories of homeowners violently assaulted after opening their doors to individuals holding a FEDEX or UPS package. Often these offenders are wearing uniforms that are almost identical to those of legitimate mail carriers. I can go down to the local Walmart and find a chocolate brown button-up shirt, matching shorts, and a brown baseball hat in thirty minutes. If I put that on, have a clipboard in one hand and a package in the other, would you open your door for me?

There has recently been a spike in home burglaries and violent home invasion assaults with offenders dressed as FEDEX or UPS delivery personnel. If you're not expecting a package and someone comes to your door with a package in hand, do not open it. If they ask for a signature, tell them to leave the package at their warehouse and you will pick it up later; or call their office to confirm they do indeed have a package delivery for you.

It is in these situations when you need to listen to your "gift of fear." If your senses are telling you something is not right, listen to them carefully. If possible, always look for the FEDEX, UPS, US Postal Service truck to help verify the person at your door is truly there for a delivery. Furthermore, most doors have peepholes; if yours does not, have one installed and use it. Never open the door for someone that you do not know.

More Home Security Tricks

In addition to motion lighting, stronger doors, harder locks, and alarm systems, there are other inexpensive things you can do to make the burglars look for a softer target.

If you have a dog, that's great. If it is a small dog, one that never stops barking at the sound of someone at the door, that's even better. If you do not have a dog, pretend that you do. Purchase a large dog bowl and put it on your front or rear porch. If someone is casing your home, they will see the dog bowl and consider looking for a different target.

I am a big fan of home security systems, especially those that automatically call the police when activated. Whether you have a security system or not, a security sign posted in your front lawn is a huge deterrent to would-be robbers. Also having window stickers indicating you have a home security system is another means of thwarting would-be thieves.

The last thing a burglar or thief wants is to be caught on camera as they rummage through your home. Installing security cameras in and around your home is a great way to secure your property. In today's modern world we now have doorbells with fish-eye cameras that feed the video and audio straight to your smartphone. You can observe and talk to the person at your front door even if you are a continent away. However, if a camera security system is not in your budget, buy a fake camera security system. These plastic, fake cameras mount near your door and even have a small battery-operated blinking red light. If a thief is casing your home and sees a red blinking light on what looks like a camera, he is not going to take time to consider whether the camera is real or not.

Criminals may be lazy, but they aren't necessarily stupid.

In post-arrest interviews of burglars, many admit to heading straight to the master bedroom once they gained entry into your home. They know the master bedroom is where most people store their cash and jewelry. Be smarter than the criminals! Be creative about where you store your cash and other valuables in your home.

Purchase spray cans that have a fake bottom to store extra cash. Buy some hollowed-out books to store jewelry. These storage books can be easily made using a simple box cutter and hollowing out some pages in an old, hardback novel. False bottom containers can be made by simply using a can opener on the bottom of a can of beans, for example. Remove the bottom part of the can, empty the contents and place your valuables or cash in the can, replace the bottom and put it on the shelf with your other canned vegetables. The can will be unrecognizable as a storage container for valuables, and a criminal is not going to waste time going through your pantry or cupboard looking for cash.

Since the master bedroom is the target for most burglars, and we know they want to spend as little time as possible in your home, it's not a bad idea to leave a little money and some cheap jewelry in plain sight to make the thief think he has gotten his loot, and leave.

Developing a Safety Plan

Just as active shooter response requires advance planning, so does home security. This means developing a plan of action with your family that addresses common dangers, including house fires, natural disasters, and home invasions.

"In a time of crisis, the time for planning has passed." I am not sure who came up with this quote, but I use it often when closing out my lectures on personal security, situational awareness, and active shooter response. This quote is also true for a home invasion. Do not wait until you are in the middle of the most horrific event of your life to make a plan of action. Make a plan with your family today. Communicate that plan; rehearse the plan; and review it with your family yearly. A good home defense plan should be quick, simple, and decisive. Remember, you will be under extraordinary stress and fear, so the plan has to be easy to follow.

One of the first considerations in developing a plan is whether or not you have children and if so, where are their bedrooms located in relation to your room? Many homes have the master bedroom downstairs while the kids' rooms are upstairs. This creates a bit of a challenge. Other homes are designed with the master bedroom at one end of the hallway while the other rooms are located on the opposite end. Your plan will be quite different and much simpler if you live alone or with your spouse.

Second, you need to determine where you are going to "hard point" or "shelter-in-place." The shelter-in-place is used to consolidate your family in one room, which has been enhanced (detailed below) to keep intruders out and you safe inside, while waiting for police to arrive. Always remember, if you can safely get out of your home and to a neighbor's, do so without hesitation. Your first course of action should always be "get off the X"; in this case, it is your home. If you cannot get your family safely out of the home, your next course of action should be get them all in one room and prepare to defend yourself if necessary.

Your "hard point" should be a bedroom or a bathroom, preferably one with a window for easy escape. You can also add a deadbolt cylinder lock on the door. These are inexpensive and easy to install. The extra lock could provide you with time to escape and for the police to arrive. In this bedroom or bathroom, you should pre-stage it with a prepaid flip phone, with 911 programmed into the number one key—press the number 1 and it auto-dials 911. This phone should also be plugged in at all times so it's always charged. You might not have time or remember to grab your personal cellphone off the nightstand as you run to your "hard point" or safe room. If it's on the second floor, the room should have a portable, collapsible, escape ladder to get out of your home and run to a neighbor's house. Stage a small medical kit, flashlight, and some kind of weapon in this room. The weapon could be a baseball bat, screwdriver, hammer, knife, or pepper spray. If you have a vehicle that you park in your garage or on the street, you should keep a spare key fob in the room as well. Once you are safely in the room, press the panic button on the key fob to initiate your car's alarm. This noise alone could scare the intruder away.

If you live alone or with your spouse, your home defense plan is fairly simple. You should go to your bathroom or master bedroom and lock the door and call 911. Then set off the car alarm and grab your weapon and be prepared to use it. Yell out to the intruder, "I have a gun and I have called the police, and if you step one foot into this room I am going to shoot you!" Whether you have a gun or not is irrelevant. The point is to make the intruder think you have a gun. The next sound you'll probably hear is that of running feet and the front door slamming behind the intruder. When you call 911, tell the operator who you are, where you are (both the address of the house and your location in the house), and that you need immediate police response, and try to stay on the line to continue to provide information on the situation as it develops.

If you have children, you need to get them together in your safe room. Then you either stay with them, or take a tactical position inside your home. A tactical position could be at the top of the stairway, or down a long hallway. It should be some place where you can observe the intruder to see if he attempts to get near you or your family. It needs to be a position that is defensible. The top of a stairway is a natural "choke point" and is advantageous to you if you are armed. The challenge may be how to get from your bedroom to the children's rooms to rally them, and bring them to the safe room. I cannot tell you how to do this without conducting an on-site assessment of your home. You must devise a plan to get safely from your room to all the other rooms, dependent upon the design of your home.

There are numerous stories of how young children have called 911 and saved the lives of parents or siblings. Make sure your child knows how to call 911 and can recite his name and address at a very early age. I recommend you role-play with your neighbor or friend posing as the 911 operator. The purpose is to teach your child how to use the phone to call for help, and when to call for emergency assistance.

Always have a list of contact names and numbers posted for your children to use in the event of an emergency. These numbers should include family members, a close neighbor who can come to your home immediately, and work numbers. Keep these posted in a convenient spot where even small children can read it.

Practice "home evacuation drills" with your children. Be sure they know all the ways to get out of the house, including break-ing a window and climbing out. In a house fire, seconds can be the difference between survival and death. Draft an evacua-tion plan and practice it with your family both in daylight and darkness. Draw a floor plan of your home on a large piece of paper and have your children show you how they would evacuate. Have them provide an alternate route in the event the primary exit is blocked by flames or debris. Teach your children to stay low during a fire and to crawl on their hands and knees to avoid the smoke. Teach them how to tell if a fire is on the other side of a closed door by using the back of their hand to feel for heat along the crack at the bottom and on the door handle.

If they have a bathroom attached to their room, show them how wet towels should be placed over the head, mouth, and nose before evacuating in a smoke-filled environment. Be sure to establish a meeting spot outside the home, where everyone is to meet once they have evacuated.

Finally, here is my most important piece of advice: put a flashlight and a whistle in your child's nightstand, or hang it on their door knob. A good flashlight will help them find their way outside, and a loud whistle will allow you or first responders to locate them quickly if they're unable to get out.

Staying Safe in Your Car

Car safety is one of the most important and often most ignored aspects of "staying safe," as carjacking is one of the fastest growing crimes in America. Vehicles have become much more difficult to steal with the newer cars having smart keys with chips imbedded in them. As a result, it is easier for criminals to steal the car directly from you, with your keys in hand.

Basic Rules of Car Safety

There are a few basic rules that should become second nature to you when you get in your vehicle.

- Always **have your keys in your hand** before you reach your vehicle. As you approach, look around the car to see who or what is parked next to you.
- Once you are near your vehicle, **look into the back seat** to make sure no one is hiding there.
- When you get into the vehicle, immediately **lock your doors, start the car, and drive away**. Do not take time to put on makeup, check your email, or tune the radio. A predator may be watching you…and this is the perfect opportunity for him to jump into your passenger seat, put a gun to your head, and demand that you drive away with him. If you have to do those things, drive a mile down the road, pull over into a populated, well-lit area, and do it there.
- **Keep your doors locked.** Most carjacking's occur while you are sitting at a stoplight and an armed criminal pulls open your (unlocked) door and sticks a gun in your face and takes your car.
- **Keep your windows up.** Too many people have fallen victim to carjackings by opening their car window when someone approaches them in a parking lot, or while stopped on the side of a street or at a stoplight. Do not open your window for anyone that you don't know.
- **Turn your car off and remove the keys when you're not in the vehicle.** Many car thefts occur when the owner leaves the car running in his driveway or at the gas station and then turns his back for just a moment. It only takes a second for someone to jump into your car and drive away. The US Department of Transportation estimates that up to half of all car thefts are a result of the driver leaving the keys in the ignition or leaving the doors unlocked with the keys on the seat. Don't make

it easy for potential car thieves to steal your vehicle by leaving your doors unlocked with your keys inside.

- **Keep your gas tank at least half full at all times.** In the event of a critical incident, natural disaster, civil unrest, or when trying to evade an armed criminal, you'll need enough fuel in your car to get you away from the dangerous situation.

- **Watch the hands.** You are most vulnerable in your vehicle when you are stopped at a traffic light. Maintain good situational awareness, and if someone approaches your vehicle, be sure to check their hands. If they reach for a weapon, drive, move; get off the X. Remember, to freeze is to die, to move is to live. For this reason it is always a good tactic to stop your vehicle far enough away from the vehicle in front of you so you can see their rear tires. This will ensure you have enough room to maneuver around the vehicle and escape the area should the need arise.

Be aware of the numerous ruses or tricks criminals will use to get you to pull over and steal your vehicle and possibly take you hostage. The "bump and rob" technique is a common ploy. The criminals will hit you from behind in a fender-bender. When you get out of your vehicle to inspect the damage, they put a gun to your face and demand the keys to your car. Another common method is for one of the conspirators to stand on the side of the road—usually it's a woman—and flag down a passing motorist by pretending she has car trouble. You, as the Good Samaritan, pull over to offer assistance, and her accomplices hop out of the vehicle and demand your keys, wallet, and whatever else their depraved minds can think of. The best defense against being a victim of a carjacking is to be vigilant, be situationally aware, and "Live in the Yellow." In most instances, if you maintain situational awareness, you'll see the carjacker before he gets to your side window. Have a plan to drive away!

Actions to Take If You Are Carjacked

As previously stated, in the event you find yourself at the mercy of a criminal, your first course of action is to move! Run or drive away if possible. Do not "freeze in fear"; remember that movements save lives.

If someone does get into your car and puts a gun to your head, DO NOT DRIVE OFF WITH HIM! Instead, gun the engine and crash into anything solid, wrecking the car. Your air bag will deploy and protect you. If the criminal is in the front passenger seat or in the back seat, he will get the worst of it. As soon as the car crashes, bail out and run. This is a better option than having the police find your lifeless body in a remote location.

Another option if a carjacker gains access to your car is to immediately turn off your engine and throw the keys out a window or an opened door. By throwing your keys as far away as possible, you will have foiled the carjacker's plan to drive off with you. There is a good chance the carjacker will leave your vehicle and search for another victim. Once he starts to get out of the vehicle, immediately open your door and run away, keeping the car between you and the carjacker.

If you are being forced to get into a car, fight as if your life depended on it—it does! Use your gun, knife, tactical pen, elbows, and knees to do whatever you need to ensure you do not end up trapped in the car with the carjacker.

If you are thrown into the trunk of a car, kick out the back taillights and stick your arm out of the hole and start waving like crazy. The driver won't see you, but everybody else will. Another method to escape from a trunk of a car is to get on all fours, arch your back up like a cat, and push hard into the truck lid.

The force should be enough to pop the trunk open. Lastly, you can often escape from the trunk by kicking the rear seat panels. Many will fold down and you can escape through the car's interior.

Should you ever need to break your car window, remember it must be done on the corners of the window where the glass tension is at its tightest. Strike the corner of the window hard with your tactical pen, the high heel of a woman's shoe, or a special window punch tool (specifically designed to break windows). I have seen very large, well-muscled men strike the center of a car window with a baseball bat and have the bat bounce back and hit them in the face without breaking the window. The side windows in almost every vehicle are made with safety glass. Once you break the integrity of the glass, it will completely shatter and fall in little crumbs. There will be no sharp shards of glass to cut you.

What to Do If You Are Kidnapped, Abducted, or Taken Hostage

A kidnapping occurs somewhere in the world every ten minutes; only about 10 percent are reported to authorities. As an American traveling abroad, you are a potential target for kidnapping—understand and recognize this as a threat every time you travel overseas. Kidnapping is a significant "weapon of influence" and source of funding for criminals and terrorists from South America to Southeast Asia to Africa.

Situational awareness is critical in preventing you from becoming a victim of a kidnapping. Your abductors will have to conduct surveillance on you to determine your patterns and your locations in order to formulate a plan to take you. If you're maintaining constant vigilance, you will probably notice these people who are watching you. If you do, notify the US Embassy, alter your routines, notify local police and hotel security staff, or consider cutting your visit short and returning home.

If you are the victim of a kidnapping, abduction, or hijacking, it is important not to stare your abductors in the eye. Direct eye contact is recognized as intimidation, and most abductors will react with greater hostility if they perceive you to be a threat. Your actions in the first sixty minutes of the abduction are critical to your survival and possible escape.

In those initial moments of the hostage situation, your abductor may be nervous and perhaps even scared. Although he has probably planned this out, the reality of what's happening and the number of variables and unknowns may make him very edgy. Do everything he asks of you, be compliant and non-threatening. Then wait. Wait for him to drop his guard, look away, or make a mistake, and then make your move—striking him in the most vulnerable areas. The most vulnerable area on every mammal, including human beings, is the eyes. Remember, "If violence is the last resort, you better be good at it." When you attack the eyes, your goal is for complete destruction. You are not trying to inflict pain; you are trying to completely blind or incapacitate your abductor.

Use every ounce of energy in your body to inflict the most amount of damage in order to ensure your escape.

The best time to counter-attack is during this initial phase of the abduction. After about five to eight minutes, the kidnapper will suffer from an adrenaline dump, which will drain him physically and emotionally. Your abductor may be exhausted from the adrenaline dump and will be slower to react to your violent counter-assault. This is also the time when you are at your strongest. You are most likely well fed and hydrated at this point. This will change if your abduction lasts more than a day or two. Use the fact that you are at your strongest to the best advantage. This is not the time to be timid or compliant. Fight, strike, gouge, and kick as if your life depended on it. Remember, you are not striking your kidnapper to inflict pain; you are violently striking your enemy to inflict traumatic injury in order completely incapacitate or kill your opponent.

Be advised, however, that you are at significant risk of injury if you fight back and attempt to escape. You have to weigh that information against the risk of being held captive for days, weeks, months, or even years. Your survival mindset should guarantee you have no issues about using extreme violence to affect your escape.

After 24 Hours

If you are unable to fight your way to freedom in the first twenty-four hours, then you'll need to put on an act of compliance. This is just an act. Be submissive, use humor if you can to make yourself more human in your abductor's eyes, be a low-maintenance hostage. The reason you want to "act" submissive and compliant is so your captors will not think you are a threat or escape risk. While you are acting compliant, you are always assessing the situation and looking for that moment when your captor lowers his guard and provides you an avenue of escape. Once you see that opportunity, run and keep running. Do not escape and then hide; chances are your abductor will find you. Run to the nearest area where people can be found, then scream for help.

How to Get Out of Restraints

The four most common items used to restrain someone are duct tape, zip ties, rope, and handcuffs—in that order. All four of these are relatively easy to escape from if you know a few simple tricks. Most people give up once their hands and feet are tied. They have systematically been taken out of the fight because they do not know how to escape from these simple restraints. Knowing a few basic skills will give you confidence if you are ever abducted and thrown into the trunk of a car or a darkened room.

Duct Tape. Duct tape is the restraint of choice for most criminals. It is cheap, easy to find, and provides a quick and easy way to restrain someone. In my Travel Security Training Courses I always choose one of the largest guys in the room. I bring them up and wrap their wrists in twelve to fifteen wraps of duct tape. Then I ask them to try and get out. The laughter in the room is spontaneous as they pull and pull on the tape, use their teeth, or attempt to twist their hands free. It is actually very tiring and eventually they give up.

The key to getting out of duct tape is all about technique.

If you are being duct-taped with your hands bound in front of your body, press your elbows and forearms together to create a tight bond at your wrists—it makes breaking the tape much easier. To break free, raise your hands high above your head; then in one quick, forceful motion, pull your arms down to your sides while expanding your chest out. Pretend you are trying to drive your elbows to the small of your back as you swiftly bring your arms down. You'll be surprised how easy it is to break free from your restraints.

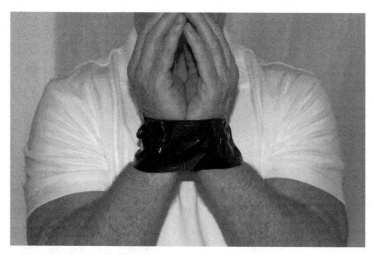

Figure 9 Escape from Duct Taped Wrists

You must practice this technique. If you are having a hard time breaking free, it is most likely because you not pulling your arms down past your hips and driving your elbows to the small of your back, while pushing your chest out. The motion is fast, swift, quick and violent!

The most common question I get asked in my training courses is, "What if they tape my hands behind my back?" Good question. In all likelihood, your abductor will tape your hands in front of you because it is simpler, faster, and allows him to grab your taped hands more easily in order to control you. However, should you have your hands duct-taped behind you, all you need to find is sharp, ninety-degree corner, such as a wall, table top, or the side of a chair. Place your taped hands in the middle of the edge and move your hands back and forth in a sawing motion until the corner cuts through your restraints.

Zip Ties. The second most common form of restraint used by criminals is zip ties. These plastic devices are also cheap, easy to use, and very accessible. Like duct tape, zip ties are fairly easy to defeat if you know the proper technique. Don't let restraints such as zip ties, duct tape, or even handcuffs drain you psychologically. Know that your freedom is just one simple technique away.

The proper technique used to defeat zip ties is very similar to getting out of duct tape. While being zip-tied, you want to keep your forearms together (as you were instructed to do with duct tape). Once your captor is out of sight, you'll want to rotate the "locking mechanism" of the zip ties to a position on top of your wrists, centered between your two hands. The easiest way to rotate the zip tie is by using your teeth.

Once you have the locking mechanism positioned on top of your wrists and centered between your two hands, use the same technique to break free as with duct tape. Raise your bound hands above your head and with one swift, aggressive action, pull your arms down to your hips, driving your elbows to the small of your back, while pushing your chest outward. The locking mechanism on the zip tie should break open and free your hands.

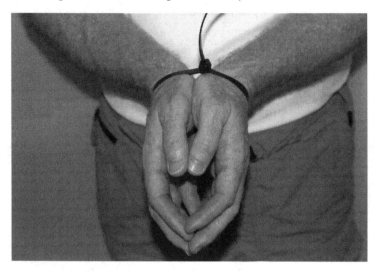

Figure 10 Proper Placement of Zip Ties for Escape

Truth be told, escaping zip ties does take a bit more strength and finesse than it does with duct tape. You have to get the right angle when you pull your arms down and apart as your expand your chest out.

Another method of escaping zip ties is by using 550-cord, also known as paracord. All zip ties are made from plastic, and all plastic can melt with heat or friction. Use paracord as a replacement for your shoelaces. Paracord comes in a variety of colors so you can match almost any shoelace. Untie one of your shoes leaving the shoelace (paracord) still attached, but have enough slack to put the paracord through your zip-tied hands. While still bending over, use your other foot to stand on the loose end of the paracord shoelace. Keep the paracord tight, one end attached to your untied shoe, the other end under your other foot, with your zip tie underneath the paracord shoelace.

Rapidly move your hands back and forth in a sawing motion so that the paracord cuts through the plastic zip-tie.

Additionally, any sharp corner can be used to generate heat and cut through the plastic zip tie as well. It may take a little longer, but ultimately by creating friction the resulting heat will overcome this restraint.

Rope. Although not as common as duct tape or zip ties, rope is often used by criminals to restrain their victims. The trick or technique to defeat rope is found in the positioning of your arms as you are being tied up. Unlike being bound with duct tape or zip ties, you do NOT want to keep your forearms together. You want to create as much space as possible through your bent wrists as you keep your elbows out.

After you have been tied (keeping your elbows out) and your captor is out of sight, straighten your arms, pointed away from your chest, palms together—pointing both hands in front of you. With your palms together and your arms straight, start moving your hands back-and-forth, as if you are trying to warm up your palms using friction. Use your flat hands as shims and ultimately you will be able to pull one of your hands free from the rope restraint. This technique works better on thicker rope. Also be aware you'll probably suffer from rope burns while doing this, but the alternative of being held captive is much worse!

It is also possible to escape a rope restraint by using 550-cord. Again, using a quick sawing motion, paracord can cut through rope. It is not as easy as cutting through plastic zip ties, but it can be done.

Remember, the purpose of this information is to get you to "stay in the fight"; to never give up; to maintain that survival mindset which tells you, "You are never defeated." All restraints can be overcome. These are just some of the methods to do so.

Handcuffs. Handcuffs are not the criminal's first choice of restraints. They are not as cheap or as easy or accessible as the other restraints mentioned above. However, it is important to know how to break out of handcuffs should you need to do so.

The easiest way to get out of handcuffs is to use a handcuff key! That is why I have handcuff keys duct taped to the inside of every one of my belts at the center of my back. Since they are universal, one key works on most handcuffs. If I am handcuffed with my hands behind my back, I have easy access to a key. Additionally, I have handcuff keys hidden in my shoes and boots. I always have at least two handcuff keys on me, and sometimes more if I am traveling overseas. These keys can be purchased online for very little, and hiding them in your clothing is always a good idea, especially if you're a frequent foreign traveler. As a side note, handcuff keys are not on the TSA's list of forbidden items.

Want to know a magician's secret? The Great Houdini became the greatest escape artist ever because he knew how to pick a simple lock, and he knew the importance of having shims on hand. Handcuffs are amazingly simple to get out of with a simple shim!

You can create a shim by simply using a child's hair barrette. Secreting a barrette in your hair, along the top of your neck, is an easy way to ensure you always have a means and mechanism to get out of handcuffs should the need arise. I know my wife and daughters always travel with a barrette hidden somewhere in their hair. I also keep barrettes clipped to the top of my pants, under my belt. This provides easy access regardless of how I am handcuffed.

This type of barrette can be purchased at any drug store, Walmart, Target, and most grocery stores. I'm talking about the cheapest, smallest barrette you can find. You are ultimately going to break this barrette and use it as a shim to defeat your handcuffs. This, too, is quite simple but does require some practice.

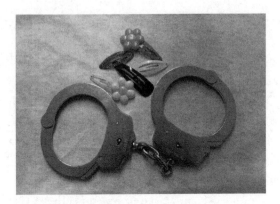

Figure 11 Various Types of Hair Clips for Handcuff Escape

First, break the barrette and remove the middle piece. Just keep bending it back and forth and the thin metal will break away fairly easily. You can discard this small center piece. The remaining part of the barrette becomes your shim. Now, break off the larger, rounded head of the barrette by continually bending the piece over and back until it breaks off, which can then be discarded. You should have two, thin pieces of metal remaining, attached by a small pivot pin; each side will be approximately one and a half inches long, forming a V. This is your shim!

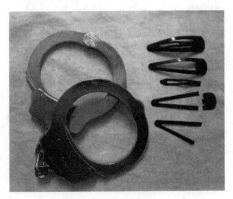

Figure 12 How to Break the Hair Clip for Escape

Look closely at the handcuffs, and you will see where the teeth of the outer part of the handcuffs slip inside the base of the cuffs, where it joins an opposing set of teeth—this locks the cuffs and is the location where you want to insert your handmade shim.

Slip the shim into the area where the teeth of the handcuffs are inserted into the base of the handcuff. You may have to tighten the cuffs as you push the shim in as deep as it can go. While pushing the shim into the slot between the teeth and cuff base, you may hear a click or two of the handcuffs as they are pushed tighter, but this is okay. Once the shim is fully inserted, you should be able to reverse the teeth out of the base while holding the shim in place. Do not let the shim back out as you reverse the cuff teeth out of the base.

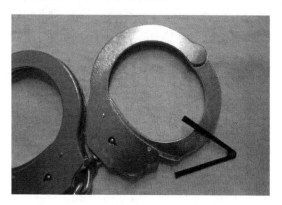

Figure 13 This is the Shim to use for Escape

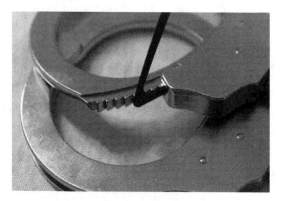

Figure 14 Proper Placement of the Shim

Having the skills to break out of restraints is empowering, and they will greatly increase your chances of survival if you are ever abducted. The techniques and skills described above are not difficult, but they do require a bit of practice. There are dozens of videos on the internet showing exactly how to defeat these restraints. I recommend you watch them and practice with your spouse, kids, co-workers, and friends.

Daughter's Date Night

A few years ago my middle daughter came home from college with a sorority sister during her spring break. One night she and her sorority sister met two young men when they went to a local honky-tonk (yes, we have those in Texas). A few days later, they called and asked my daughter if she and her friend would like to go see a Texas Rangers baseball game. My daughter asked me if that would be okay and after a few routine questions, I said, "sure."

Two days went by and I came home from work early to meet these men. The girls were still getting ready when the doorbell rang and I answered the door. I intentionally did not remove my FBI badge, weapon, spare magazines, and handcuffs. When I opened the door, I received the exact response I was hoping for–fear!

With a big smile I said, "Oh, didn't my daughter tell you I was an FBI special agent?" They asked me a few questions about being a special agent, and they were very polite. Then I told them I didn't know their last names, and I wouldn't be good father if I allowed my daughter to go out with men I didn't know. So, I asked to see their driver's licenses. They hesitated briefly and I said, "I'm serious." When they handed me their licenses, I took out my cellphone and snapped a quick photo. I told them it was my duty as a father to protect my daughter, and I would never allow her to get into another man's car without knowing who was driving.

When the girls came into the living room, my daughter knew instantly something was amiss. She looked at me and said, "Dad, what did you do?" I smiled and said, "Nothing. I'm just chatting with your dates." As the four left and got into their vehicle, I followed them outside. Then, I took out my phone again and took a photograph of the car and license plate, and told them to have a good time. My daughter was a bit embarrassed, but deep inside she knew I was only trying to protect her and her best friend.

Do not be afraid to take a photo of your child's date and their driver's license and car. Your child may be angry with you initially, and will probably be a bit embarrassed, but they will know their date is fully informed not to mess around!

I later learned that after they got into the car, one of the guys said, "Your dad is a pretty intense guy." My daughter replied, "Yeah, I know. He loves me!"

Chapter 6
COMMUNITY SECURITY (CHURCHES & SCHOOLS)

Nothing strikes a deeper fear into the soul of our nation than a mass shooting at a school or house of worship. These incidents have become all too common, and we have kicked that can down the street far too long. It is time to come to grips with the fact that evil does exist, and our children, as well as churchgoers, are often the targets of such evil. We need to stop such shootings!

School Security

I truly believe that the increase in school violence is a cultural issue. School shootings did not occur thirty or forty years ago despite the fact many kids brought guns to school in the back of their pickup trucks. These rifles were brought on to school grounds (locked in their vehicles) so the student could go on an evening hunt after class. It is also true the percentage of homes with guns (approximately 42 percent) has not increased over the last several decades (Statista 2017). So, what has changed?

Is the fact our children are being raised in day-care centers instead of at home with a parent having a negative impact on our kids? Are we overprescribing antidepressants and ADHD medicine for our children? Have the court systems become a revolving door for repeat offenders? Have violent movies and video games desensitized our kids to violence? Are any of these at fault, or is it a culmination of all these things? Whatever the reason, the true answer to school violence is through cultural changes. In my opinion, our culture has devalued human life, and the change has affected our children. Has the sanctity of life and respect for our fellow man been marginalized through legalized abortion, pornography, and violent movies and video games? Cultural changes can take an entire generation before taking effect. What can we do now, as teachers, parents, students, and as a society, to make our schools safer?

I have been interviewed on dozens of news programs, radios shows, and in print media, and I am often asked how we can address this violence. I always respond that to stop mass shootings in our nation's schools requires a multifaceted solution. One that demands innovative, out of the box thinking, money, and an unwavering commitment to counseling and training.

The current security plan for US schools is not working.

It is important to realize that there is no magic pill or one-size-fits all for securing our schools. Each school is unique. There are six-story schools in New York City, and sprawling multi-acre school campuses in Texas. The security plans for each of these schools will be entirely different. A complete paradigm shift is needed in our government, in our schools, in our students, and in their parents in order to fix this. Having the Department of Education or Homeland Security develop a nationwide active shooter response for schools is not the answer. The design, development, and implementation of a safe and effective active shooter response plan needs to be specific for each school...and that costs money.

In presenting my case on how to better secure our nation's schools, I use the White House as an example. The White House is one of the most secure structures in the world. It is aesthetically pleasing, has great curb appeal, conducts public tours for thousands of visitors daily, and yet remains secure. If we can do that to the White House, we can do it to our schools.

Providing outstanding security to our nation's schools is not impossible. It should include unobtrusive fencing, access gates, bullet-resistant glass, drop walls, hardened rooms, armed security, magnetometers, video surveillance, panic buttons, shot-location devices, a campus-wide communication network, continual training of the staff, and enhanced school counseling. I believe this holistic approach will give us safer schools. Individually these things are fairly easy to accommodate, however, as an all-encompassing security plan, the costs would be considerable for most school districts and certainly for private schools. One has to ask, "What is the price for keeping our children safe?"

Note that gun control is not listed as a necessity to secure our nation's schools. Without getting into a political debate, I believe taking away guns from law-abiding citizens and limiting their ability and constitutional right to defend themselves is senseless and wrong. However, those with mental health issues or criminal backgrounds should never be able to purchase a weapon. Armed citizens have prevented many crimes and those carrying a concealed weapon have saved many lives (Elder 2018).

One of the biggest issues pertaining to security in today's school systems is whether or not to have a vulnerability assessment completed. School administrators are concerned that if they have a comprehensive security or threat assessment done, they will not have the money to implement the recommendations, which would then put the school at financial risk should a shooting occur.

After the 2018 Valentine's Day shooting at Marjory Stoneham Douglas High School, in Parkland, Florida, where seventeen students and faculty were killed and another seventeen were wounded, there were calls to make schools a "hardened target"—for example, by arming teachers. I believe it is necessary to have an "intervention capable response" or an "armed response" on the school grounds. Whether it is an armed teacher program, or hiring armed security guards, there needs to be an armed response on-site. There is an old shooter's proverb that states: "The only way to stop a bad man with a gun is with a good man with a gun." If a psychotic mass murderer goes to a school and starts shooting with his brand of hate and violence, the only way to eliminate the threat is to neutralize the shooter. It may take a firearm to do this. It is important to remember the average time of an active shooter event is eight minutes, while the average police response time is twelve minutes. Having an armed response on campus is critical. We must understand, during most active shooter events, the police will not arrive in time to help.

Whether employing an armed teacher program or using armed security guards, both require tactical training, surgical shooting skills, and an understanding of the body's response to high-stress, high-threat encounters. A continual training program is needed in order to maintain this necessary skill set, and this takes time, commitment, mindset, and money.

But, as we learned from the Douglas High School (Parkland, Florida) active shooter event, having an armed officer isn't necessarily going to stop the killing. Although the inactions of the school resource officer assigned to Douglas High School was far from the norm, it does show that the human element is fallible. Not every sworn police officer (or security officer) has the "warrior mindset" with the courage to run toward the gunfire, as evident in the Parkland, Florida, incident. I recommend every school resource officer, armed teacher, and school security guard read books such as *On Combat*, *The Gift of Fear*, or *When Violence is the Answer* in order to understand the body's response to high-stress and deadly encounters. These books will not guarantee the reader will develop that warrior mindset, but it will enlighten them to reconsider their choice of being an armed response in a school and whether they have the fortitude and the will to run to the gunfight when required to do so.

Having magnetometers (metal detectors), locked doors, and armed officers is not the solution to stop a determined individual from getting a weapon into a school. It is effective, but not 100 percent effective. We need to start thinking outside the box and in a more comprehensive manner about **prevention**. The training, manpower and equipment required for a **reaction** are easy! Prevention is the hard part.

I firmly believe the only way to stop, or *react*, to an active shooter is with an armed response. That being said, I also believe there is a lot we can do to *prevent* a disgruntled student with a gun from wanting to murder his fellow students—mainly by increasing the number of school counselors, training them to recognizing pre-incident indicators to violence, and mandating that those students determined to be "high risk" participate in counseling, along with their parents.

Preventing School Violence

If we are really talking about prevention, my thought is that we need to look at school violence as a mental health issue and go for the public health approach. I am not a psychologist, nor do I pretend to be. However, I feel that if the school counseling programs were enhanced and we took a good look at both bullying and discrimination in our schools, we would find we would be better able to identify potential threats (high-risk individuals) and take specific action on those threats. It was no surprise to students and faculty at Douglas High School who the shooter was once he was identified. Could the Douglas High School shooter have been rehabilitated had he and his parents been required to attend counseling? Could the shooting have been prevented with a more aggressive anti-bullying campaign on campus? Had the shooter's mental health been better evaluated, would this have prevented the killing? Answers we will never know, but improving our school counseling programs may be the first step to mitigate this current trend.

Most people understand the term "corporate culture"; it is the pervasive values, beliefs, and attitudes that characterize a company and guides its practices. A school's culture is similar. It is based on the relationships between students, teachers and parents. It is affected by the school's approach to discipline, behavioral issues, and the availability and accessibility of school counselors. Cultivating a school's culture which addresses the negative aspects, such as bullying, discrimination, exclusion-based social cliques, threats, loners, and poor academic performers, as well as the positive characteristics like social norms, manners, respect, and school pride, is difficult but essential. The question remains, How do schools change their culture when the average student-to-school-counselor ratio is 482-to-1—nearly double the 250-to-1 ratio recommended by The American School Counselor Association (Fuschillo 2018)? Those are unacceptable numbers. Our prisons have far better prisoner-to-counselor ratios.

While school counselor's core function is to shepherd students into either college or career, counselors are also responsible for helping manage students' social-emotional health throughout their school years. Yet only a fraction of children that exhibit symptoms of a mental health disorder receive help.

Professionals—such as a school psychologist—dedicated to addressing mental health issues are in short supply in school districts across the nation and often work across two or more schools. This means that the average school counselor is often the first point of contact for addressing bullying, discrimination, and other students' social-emotional needs.

Why is school culture so important? Because how a school responds to troubled students can very well have a big impact on the actions of those students. The kids who bring weapons to school are the same kids most likely to report being bullied or threatened. They may be fearful of gang violence and feel the need to protect themselves, or they may be picked on or ostracized. A 2015 study in the journal *Pediatrics* showed the kids who bring weapons to school often are the same kids who reported being victimized. The study concluded: "Pediatricians should recognize that VoBs (Victims of Bullying), especially those who have experienced one or more indicators of peer aggression in conjunction, are at substantially increased risk of weapon carrying" (Pham et al.).

If schools devote resources to aggressively address bullying, threats, discrimination, and harassment, there is a better chance those schools will be more successful in identifying a conflict before it gets out of hand.

Along with enhanced counseling, school administrators need to develop and instill a "Safe-to-Tell" program where students feel comfortable talking to adults, teachers, or counselors. We know from after action reports on school shootings that a majority of the time other students had heard of the pending assault. Kids talk! Kids boast! Kids hear! It is essential to have a program that makes it easy and anonymous for students to report on those kids who bring weapons into a school, or who are overheard discussing a planned attack.

A quick and easy way to have a reporting portal is to install a toll-free, anonymous, no-caller ID 800 number. This will provide students an anonymous means to report suspicious behavior, bullying, or threats to the school. There are dozens of other communication apps and networks that have similar functions. Do a little research and find one that best fits your school's needs.

A National Center for Education Statistics report showed among students ages 12–18, there were about 749,400 victimizations (theft and nonfatal violent victimization) at school and 601,300 victimizations away from school. During this time, 10 percent of public school teachers reported being threatened with injury by a student, and 6 percent reported being physically attacked by a student (Musu-Gillette 2017). If a student, or bullying victim, has a safe, anonymous way to report these victimization incidents, faculty and law enforcement can then address it directly with the offender.

Threat Assessments

How to approach the offender? Let me give you an example of what the US Secret Service does when they receive an anonymous call detailing a threat to the president of the United States.

My younger brother is a retired, 25-year US Secret Service (USSS) special agent. He is highly trained and an expert at quickly identifying who is a potential threat. He bases this on years of experience and excellent training. When the USSS identifies an individual who is a potential threat from a confidential source (informant), by a threatening letter, social media post, or the crazed ranting of a mentally unstable individual, they conduct a threat assessment on that individual. The USSS then talks to the reporting source (if known), conducts database checks, visits with neighbors and friends, and visits the workplace and determines if the person in question owns any weapons or has any special skills or military training. They delve deep into this person's past and his current life to determine whether he poses a real threat. I recommend school districts implement this as part of their security plan and do the same type of threat assessment when they are informed of a potential threat.

A threat assessment team consisting of the principal, school counselor, a selected teacher, and the school security director can develop a plan to talk to those involved, as well as their friends, neighbors and family to determine if the threat is genuine. If so, law enforcement, the district attorney's office, mental health specialists, and school administrators can then take the appropriate steps to counsel, suspend, or, if necessary, incarcerate the high-risk individual.

Training and communications are the essential items needed for any school security plan. The teachers, custodial crew, cafeteria staff, and administration personnel all need to be trained in how to respond in the event of an active shooter. Every staff member and teacher needs to feel as if they are the most important part in the security plan. Every employee needs to have a burning desire to ensure the security plan is communicated and practiced.

Secondly, a school-wide communication and monitoring network needs to be implemented. This system can be as simple as hand-held radios for each teacher along with a monitored CCTV system. It could encompass cell phone applications that immediately convey critical information to a designated group. Or, it could be as extensive as social media monitoring, geo-fencing, perimeter cameras with facial and object recognition capabilities, and state-of-the-art "shot detection or localization" software, which instantly identifies the location of gunfire and transfers the information to any number of cell phones. Real-time shot localization information would enable teachers, staff, police dispatch, and armed security on campus to immediately know *where* the shots were fired. Some systems can identify if the shot was fired from a handgun or a rifle—critical information for responding police units. Using this information a teacher can instantly determine whether they should evacuate the school or shelter in place, and the armed response would know the exact location of the threat.

These high-tech solutions implemented into emergency response and crisis management plans will eliminate confusion in the initial response to an active shooter. These systems can provide immediate situational awareness to everyone involved and allow for a more informed response. These systems integrate the school's vulnerability assessment with:

- Monitoring of social media and the dark net, looking for offensive or threatening content
- Identification of individuals through facial recognition on over 2000 databases, or compared against a list of those that have been identified as a threat
- Prevention (weapon detection) via magnetometers or other available high-end detection systems able to detect certain metal alloys and gunpowder
- Mitigation with shooter localizations systems which instantly detect, identify, and communicate the location of the shooter both indoors and out
- Notification through communication networks, which quickly and cost effectively combines information gathering, situational awareness, and secure messaging capabilities

Even with high-tech security solutions, the basic requirement is still the capability of every teacher to be able to quickly and confidently lock their classroom to prevent the shooter from gaining access. A locking mechanism for every door must be present, along with ballistic glass and the ability to cover the window so the shooter cannot see inside the classroom. The locking mechanism must be easy to engage and require little to no fine-motor skills (which are severely diminished during high-stress, critical incidents). The ability to quickly and safely shelter in place is essential in every school active shooter security plans.

Being able to shelter in place is important; however, the key to surviving any shooting incident is to move! Run! Get out if at all possible! It is very important to remember, hiding does not work! In every school-shooting event, I see social media posts showing children hiding underneath their school desks. The image of frightened students hiding under plastic desks has to stop. Those desks are neither bulletproof nor good hiding spots. By hiding, you are only making yourself an easier target for massacre. In the rare instance you cannot run away from the threat ("Get off the X") and you are forced to shelter-in-place, do not attempt to hide. Lock the door, turn out the lights, and look for ways to defend yourself. Break off the leg of a chair and use it as a blunt-force baton; grab the fire extinguisher off the wall to use as an improvised weapon; find a pair of scissors, a screwdriver, or a pen—all which can be used to stop the killer with a well-placed, violent assault to the shooter's eyes or throat.

The first step to prevention is to train our teacher how to properly respond to an active shooter event. If we equip the teachers with good training and techniques in what to do, we can help prevent future deaths. Having awareness and preparedness on how to respond, the "what to do," will provide the teachers with both confidence and a peace of mind should they encounter a shooter at their school. It is the not knowing what to do that causes the unnecessary fear and anxiety.

Teachers need to be taught to stop directing their kids to hide under the desk, period. They are doing their students a disservice by instructing them to do so. I am a firm believer if you can run, do so. Remove yourself from the kill zone. Exit the building and keep moving until you find a safe place to barricade and call the police. If, in the rare instance you find yourself where you cannot exit the building, you are unable to barricade the door, and the shooter enters your room, then violence is your only solution.

> "If violence is the last resort, you better be good at it."
> —Greg Shaffer

At this moment your survival mindset is what will keep you (and your students) alive. Your mental capacity to inflict lethal force will save your life. In fact, now that you have read this book, you will have been in this exact situation hundreds of times, rehearsing it in your mind, developing a plan and picturing yourself defeating this killer. You now know the only way to survive this encounter is to use the very same tool your attacker is trying to use against you—violence. At this juncture, you are not "defending yourself"; you are incapacitating an active shooter. Attempting to use your social skills to de-escalate the situation won't work. You are not going to stop the killing by being polite, kind, or friendly. The only way the killing stops, the only way you can survive, is if you use more violence than the shooter.

The first time you devise a plan on what to do and how to respond to an active shooter should not be the moment it is happening in your classroom. This worst-case scenario needs to be rehearsed in your mind over and over again, so if that day ever comes, you will know exactly what to do.

Items Everyone Should Have in Their Desk Drawer

I conduct a lot of classroom training courses for school teachers explaining how they should respond if they are ever caught up in an active shooter event. I recommend that every teacher keep three cans of soup and a pillowcase in their desk drawer. These items would never raise suspicion and can be used as a means to break the classroom window for an escape, or they can be used as a weapon. Put the soup cans in the pillowcase and start swinging!

Other items have daily uses in a classroom that I recommend all teachers (and employees) keep in their desk drawers:

1. Hammer
2. Box Cutter
3. Screwdriver
4. Pepper Spray (if allowed) or a Tactical Pen
5. CO2 Fire Extinguisher

These five everyday items can be used for a variety of reasons and can be explained to your principal, supervisor, or boss. Having a few tools in your desk drawer is not going to set off any alarms or cause anyone to call security thinking you're a risk. At the same time, these items in the hands of you and your students, or co-workers, could make a difference in a life or death situation. These items make very capable weapons to defeat almost any violent offender.

My youngest daughter is an elementary school Special Education teacher on the East Coast. I know she keeps these items in her desk drawer and can easily justify why they are there—for hanging pictures, cutting paper, basic repairs on desks, small projects, etc. She knows these "Five Items Everyone Should Have in Their Desk Drawer" are great for everyday projects, but she is also aware how they make for even better improvised weapons.

The hammer, box cutter, and screwdriver should be obvious as to how they could be used as an improvised weapon. You use them to strike, cut, or stab your assailant until the threat has been eliminated. When choosing a pepper spray, don't buy cheap. Be sure to get a highly rated, long shooting spray. If possible, buy "Bear Spray"; it's pepper spray in a larger container and can shoot up to thirty feet. Think about how useful this could be if you sprayed it into the eyes of an armed predator. If he can't see, he can't fight!

The CO_2 fire extinguisher under your desk is there, naturally, in case of a fire. Did you know the CO_2 coming out of a fire extinguisher is minus 110 degrees Fahrenheit? Shooting a blast of CO_2 into the eyes of your active shooter will instantly freeze his corneas and he will not be able to see. After you blind your assailant with CO_2, use the heavy base of the fire extinguisher to bash in his head.

And of course, no teacher should ever be without his or her tactical pen!

Remember, "If violence is the last resort, you better be good at it!" Having a shooter in your school or office is a violent act that will only be solved with more violence. The shooter must be eliminated for the killing to stop. A horrific event for sure; but it's the only way to stop the mass killing.

Church Security

The First Baptist Church of Sutherland Springs, Texas, had only one hundred members in a town of only one thousand residents. On a sunny Texas morning in November 2017, twenty-six men, women, and children were killed and over twenty more wounded when a crazed man from a nearby town entered the small church and yelled, "Everybody die." Police found fifteen empty magazines capable of holding thirty rounds each on the floor of the church. This incident should remind us that no church is immune from potential attack. While we must resist the urge to succumb to irrational fear, churches must seriously consider the question of security, and be proactive in safeguard-ing their people. Remember, evil exists!

We are quickly learning that churches are particularly vul-nerable to the actions of murderous criminals. Motivation varies and may include robbery, domestic spillover, mental ill-ness, political differences, and religious bias. Churches, by their nature, have an open door policy during worship services, so that anyone wanting to worship God and hear the Good News of the gospel will be welcomed.

Church leaders have a duty to provide protection from poten-tially dangerous people who may be on their property, especially if they know ahead of time who these people are. The first crit-ical aspect of church security is: have a *security plan*! Once you have a plan, communicate the plan to the church staff and the congregation.

There are two primary reasons churches need to have a detailed security plan. The first is the moral obligation to ensure the safety of worshipers, staff, and property. The second is to protect the church legally against lawsuits stemming from injury caused by a person intent on killing.

Criminal acts committed by terrorists in houses of worship in other countries have used improvised explosive devices (com-monly referred to as "IEDs"), arson, small arms, assassinations, kidnapping, and chemical and biological weapons. In the United States, church attacks have been committed with handguns and rifles and are often the result of domestic spillover or mental instability and dysfunction, sometimes a mixture of all three. However, a good security plan addresses all possibilities.

History shows us that the ones most likely to do us harm are often people within our own communities who at this very moment may be nursing a grudge, or are completely bereft of conscience, and are contemplating violent actions against others.

As in school security, training and communications are the essential items needed for any church security plan. Having a reliable communication network and a high-definition CCTV surveillance system is an important asset to any church. Good communication, via radio or smartphone apps, allows the surveillance camera operator to quickly contact the church security team, provide a brief description of the situation and direct them to the threat.

I mentioned before in school security, this communication and monitoring system could be as simple as hand-held radios (with earpieces) along with a monitored CCTV system. Or it could encompass cell phone applications that immediately convey critical information to a designated group. In megachurches, the security system could include social media monitoring, geo-fencing, perimeter cameras with facial and object recognition capabilities, and state-of-the-art gunfire detection software, as previously discussed.

If the goal of the sociopath is to cause as many casualties in as short time as possible, what better place to go? A church may contain as few as twenty-five worshippers, or up to five thousand people. They are seated in a building with limited exits and the vast majority is unarmed and unable to defend themselves.

Study the following aspects a shooter might consider when targeting a church:

- Many people have assembled at a single location on a published date.
- There is easy access into the building and facilities.
- People lacking the skills and tools needed to identify or deal with potential violent criminal actors typically are at the entrances. In fact, most are there to welcome first-time visitors.

- Entrance to the church parking lot is generally unrestricted.
- Visitors unknown to members of the congregation and church staff are welcomed and invited to attend services.
- Church volunteers, workers, and maintenance staff generally do not go through background checks.
- Most churches do not have a trained security team or even a single security officer.
- While greeters and staff may have been taught to observe and report an unusual person (to recognize the anomalies in their environment), they often lack an intra-church communication system to convey their observations to key personnel. And often those key personnel are not equipped or trained on how to handle a potential violent encounter.

The best laid plans for preventing a dangerous person from entering your facility may not be enough. In the vast majority of cases, if you suspect a person poses a threat, then that person should be quietly but firmly confronted and removed. The keys to accomplishing this with minimal disruption is selecting the right time to move, knowing what to say and how to say it, and understanding that physical contact is a last resort. This may be a very tenuous and dangerous situation—removing someone who is a potential violent threat should never be taken lightly or done alone.

The dilemma for church security teams is, Do you remove the person or let them stay? Inexperienced security personnel may be tempted to storm in and drag a suspicious person away. That is generally not the right decision.

In a recent incident, a suspicious looking man walked into a Colorado church. The person had been drinking, was dirty, and was wearing a hooded parka. Church security officials also knew he was a former US Army Special Forces soldier. The security team observed him walk in and kept their eyes on him. He sat down and promptly fell asleep. The guy slept through the entire service. What's more disruptive—letting the guy sleep or making a scene? You don't make a scene if the person is not disruptive. So when the service was over, the security team approached him and told him he had to leave. This is where an experienced and trained security team comes into play.

If a disruptive person threatens violence or becomes violent, that individual needs to be quickly removed. If the person is nonviolent, the pastor may simply declare that the service is over and ask his parishioners to quietly file out of the building. While this is going on, the security team members isolate the threat and continue to ask everybody else to leave. By doing this, you are taking away his audience. I use this same technique when I am conducting dignitary protection or executive protection operations. If a protestor or heckler interrupts the program that my protectee is conducting, I remove the source of the protest. In other words, I remove my protectee. Once he is out of the room in a secured location, I have one of the staff announce he will not return until the heckler or protesters leave. You would be surprised how quickly those in the audience who want to hear the program rally to your side! The remaining attendees quickly become your ally in getting the protesters to leave.

But in more confrontational encounters, action may be necessary. When weapons are observed or when someone makes a specific threat to the church or its people, action must be taken immediately. The first thing to do is to request the person move away from the congregation. If they refuse to do so, you know this is a serious issue and potential threat.

Most churches lack the funds to equip and train an Intervention Capable Response security team. While one or more members of the congregation may indeed be skilled and capable, many variables may prevent that person from getting into a position where effective intervention is possible. It is simply not enough to own a pistol, have a license to carry, but then rely solely on inspiration and faith to take on the enormous responsibility of being an armed first responder in a house of worship.

It is important to understand that a poorly executed armed response may actually injure or cost the lives of innocent people. In addition, a poorly conceived or incompetent armed response could also subject the responder to criminal charges and expose the church itself to lawsuits. Just because the church designated someone as their official Intervention Capable Response person, or made them part of their new church security team does not imbue them with any special superhero tactical firearms skills or enforcement powers.

I recommend that anyone contemplating becoming part of their church's security team should become familiar with their state's "use of force" laws. They are likely to find that their ability to detain, arrest, or even touch another person while performing church security has not been expanded. Often civilian arrest powers within a church are limited, and the criminal penalty for false arrest or detention is punishable by a fine and jail time.

I also recommend that if you are a member of a church security team you should practice at the gun range at least once a month and shoot at least three hundred rounds per visit—minimum. If you draw your weapon and engage a threat in your church, you better hit what you are aiming at. If you miss, the chance of hitting a fellow church member is very likely. Many houses of worship are very open with large sanctuary and worship areas. What is the maximum distance from one corner of the church to the other? Are you taking shots at that distance on the gun range? Are you accurate at that distance? If you carry a gun, especially in the confines of a church, you better be absolutely sure and confident of your abilities with that weapon.

Developing a Church Security Program

Taking a 25-yard headshot with panicked parishioners running, screaming, in front of, around, and behind an active shooter is extremely risky and very difficult. In fact, there are very few shooters in the world who can consistently make that shot. If the worst happens and your church security team has to engage an active shooter inside the sanctuary, are they up to the task? Can your security team really make a 25-yard shot, on a moving target, in a crowd, with a questionable backstop? How often is your team training? Do they practice disarming techniques? Does your team practice shooting under stress? If you have ever practiced shooting at a distant moving target with a handgun, you know how difficult it is.

Another consideration is: What if the shooter is wearing body armor? Once the threat is recognized by the congregation, human nature and the physiological response to run will create a human stampede to get out of the church. How does the security team get to the shooter if they have to force their way "upstream" through a mass of frightened worshippers?

All is not lost in these scenarios, but forethought is required. Proper responses must be learned under the guidance of qualified instructors and practiced over and over. Training is the key, and training costs time and money.

The challenge for churches is to develop a plan that is neither too complex nor difficult for team members to understand, nor is so simplistic and nonspecific that team members may not know what to do when faced with a threat.

Churches interested in proactively developing a security program should consider the following:

- Designate a security director—provide him with the time and money to train his staff.
- Develop a comprehensive security and emergency response plan AND communicate that plan to all staff.

- Train staff and greeters to be additional eyes and ears for security.
- Test emergency response plans through regular exercises.
- Liaise with law enforcement, fire department, and emergency medical services.
- Develop a means of controlling access to entrances and exits during business hours and during service hours. Once the service has started, ensure only the front door remains unlocked.
- Employ a means of communication within the security team and persons assigned to observe and report.
- Consider using electronic monitoring and surveillance equipment if the facility is too large for the team to quickly observe and respond to possible threats.
- Control the hours of operation—make sure the church buildings have designated public hours with someone in the building anytime the doors are unlocked.
- Try to avoid putting employees or volunteers in situations of being alone in an empty building—there is safety in numbers.
- Invest in electronic keyed entrances. So many different people use church campus buildings that it is sometimes difficult to control who is entering a building and who has keys to the building. Electronic key cards are essential to track and control entry.
- Make sure all doors lock automatically when closing, and when possible, use steel doors and steel frames.
- Have lockdown procedures. Develop, communicate and train on lockdown procedures, especially in children's areas. Determine the best method to protect church members in the event of a threatening or unsafe situation.
- Select and train a security team.

Selected security team personnel should be thoroughly vetted with a complete background check. Training should include advance firearms skills, disarming techniques, and most importantly, how to use verbal communication to de-escalate a situation. The security team should be trained to operate in Condition Yellow and to identify threat indicators, such as persons in crowds wearing bulky clothes; unusual packages received in the mail; unattended briefcases, backpacks, or boxes; suspicious vehicles near crowds; unauthorized access to HVAC equipment; and unexpected deliveries or maintenance vehicles. The security team needs to be trained to recognize the anomalies in their environment. Once the anomaly has been identified, this information needs to be conveyed to the appropriate person, who can then dispatch additional security personnel to politely and safely approach the individual (anomaly) to ascertain whether a threat truly exists.

Members of a church security team should not only be aware of challenges associated with closing in on an active shooter in a crowd, but they should also routinely practice doing so at the gun range and in the church. Using role players in the sanctuary in a weapon-free environment can be very beneficial and add a sense of realism to the training.

My recommendation for churches interested in fielding a protective team is to first select a competent director or team leader, then assemble a team and get them properly trained. Given a choice between quickly putting together a full team of people with a lot of enthusiasm but little experience, or starting with a small team of mature people with a record of reliability and discernment, I would select the latter. The team can increase in size over time through proper vetting. If your church is not large enough for a team and there is just one person, all is not lost. If that one person does his job properly, that particular house of worship should become significantly safer.

The safety of church attendees is enhanced when trained staff and volunteers who are part of the church's overall security procedures man access points to critical areas of church. Each member of the security team should be assigned a post before, during, between, and after services.

It is preferable to keep the team leader mobile, either directing the team or in a position to move and react if necessary. I recommend that at least two team members be posted in the sanctuary during the service, one in the front and one in the back and at diagonal corners.

In larger churches with a backstage behind the pulpit, a security team member should be assigned whose primary role is to watch and protect the minister. If the church has a balcony or an upper deck, at least one team member should be posted there. There should be at least one security member assigned to the children's area, and if possible, have an off-duty, uniformed police officer outside the church during the services. This allows him to be a visible deterrent while also being able to observe people approaching the church with ill intent.

I know of one church that has a person patrolling the parking lot in an enclosed golf cart before, during, and after the services—that is a fantastic idea! If the security team is not large enough to fill all the necessary positions, the church needs to prioritize which posts are more critical and fill them accordingly.

Three Strands of Church Security

I particularly like the approach of the National Organization of Church Security and Safety Management (NOCSSM) based in Frisco, Texas, and headed by Chuck Chadwick. NOCSSM has broken church security into three layers of protection:

- Policies and procedures: These specifically address security policies, emergency actions, shelter-in-place, lockdowns, visitors, staff ID and background checks, mail screening, offering procedures, and more. These written policies should mandate compliance and not be too lengthy or complex.

- Team players: This is a carefully selected, vetted, and trained security team whose members can best be described as quiet, nonegotistical professionals. The security team needs to be familiar with use-of-force guidelines and fully understand what they can and cannot do when confronted with a variety of situations. It is my personal belief that the team should dress in the same manner as the congregation, whether suit and tie or casual dress. In larger churches, also having one or more armed and uniformed security officers or off-duty police officers on the premises indicates the church is not a soft target. Included within this second strand, but no less important, are the trained staff and volunteers, as they are often the first people to pick up on anomalies.

- Systems and equipment: Video surveillance is a wonderful tool that not only replaces trained personnel, but it can look directly at otherwise unobservable areas. Use of quality radios and earbuds permits team members to remain in contact with other team members and church staff and volunteers who may have seen something of concern. Quality radios also let the protective team communicate directly with each other. They are the quickest way for the person monitoring the security cameras to contact and direct the team in the event their presence is needed in a specific area. In addition, security systems and burglar alarms protect the premises, because not all crime happens during regular church services.

Church security is not glamorous. Normally little happens, and with time, attention wanders and complacency threatens to set in. Some team members may resign at this point, stating the job is not worth the time required, or they become unwilling to commit to being present on a specific date at a specific time. Fortunately there are always those who believe the lives of the church family should be protected against those who wish them harm, and they're willing to learn, train, and practice to defend those who cannot defend themselves.

Chapter 7
CORPORATE SECURITY

Recent statistics show that violence in the workplace is becoming more and more common. According to the US Bureau of Labor Statistics, about 5 percent of all businesses experience an incident of workplace violence each year. For larger organizations with over 1,000 employees, this rate is increased tenfold to 50 percent (2017). A 2014 FBI report found active shooter incidents in the United States now occur on an average of once a month. Of these incidents, almost half (45.6 percent) occurred at a business, while nearly a quarter (24.4 percent) occurred at schools and institutions of higher learning (FBI 2014).

In another FBI report, entitled "Study of Pre-Attack Behaviors of Active Shooters in the United States Between 2000 and 2013," Silver, Simons, and Craun (2016) note that active shooters do not bust out of extreme social isolation and commit their act of violence. Most lived with or had social interaction with other people who likely observed "pre-incident" behavioral indicators. These behavior issues could include mental health problems related to anger, paranoia, or depression; troubling levels of interpersonal conflicts; or communicated threats of violence. Active shooters almost always precede their attacks with behaviors that stir apprehension in people close to them. Having a mechanism for employee and family members to report these types of behavioral indicators are essential to mitigate the threat.

Active Shooter Response and Prevention

In December 2015, fourteen people were killed and twenty-two others were seriously injured in a terrorist attack known as the San Bernardino (California) shooting. But did you know these two terrorists also attempted to bomb the facility in which they worked? In fact, the San Bernardino facility conducted monthly active shooter training, one might be tempted to ask, Did the training work?

At many businesses, active shooter training consists of an informative lecture with too many PowerPoint slides, given by their security supervisor to employees who truly believe it will never happen to them. Many corporate active shooter drills are a waste of time and money. I should know. I have conducted hundreds of training programs at schools and businesses that have brought me in after wasting their money on a low-cost active shooter expert. My training programs empower the entire staff, from the CEO to the janitor. My courses remove the fear of not knowing what to do. We teach people how to recognize pre-incident indicators and to trust their gut instincts. My instruction includes discussions on not rationalizing their fears, and how to develop a survival mindset and situational awareness. We identify improvised weapons readily available in our client's work area. We teach all our clients that the best thing to do during an active shooter event is to run; and we teach what actions to take if you cannot run, or get yourself off the X.

Many active shooter prevention programs have the opposite effect of what they are meant to accomplish. They aren't making the employees safer; they're allowing the attackers to be more effective. Your employees do not want to be burdened by fear. They want to learn practical ways to protect themselves. Empower your employees by teaching them how to be "self-protecting." If your employees are fearful, they will make easy targets, and we know that hiding under their desks is not a viable option.

Training should be focused on modifying a person's behavioral response in the face of a threat while emphasizing that one need not live in fear of these types of events. Awareness and preparedness provide peace of mind. It's the *not knowing what to do* that causes unnecessary fear. So, what are organizations to do?

Every organization needs to have a written plan and that plan needs to be clearly communicated to all its employees. Then, that plan needs to be practiced and trained, much like the fire drill at school or lifeboat drills on a cruise ship. Only through regular, planned training exercises can workers feel prepared to face a critical incident, emergency, or active shooter event.

Statistics show that while the chances of an active shooter event are still very rare, not having a plan of action and looking the other way is not a solution to any problem, and it's one that could have deadly consequences. A strategy based on, "It won't happen to me" is a folly that could irreparably destroy a brand name or a firm's reputation and cost many lives.

The Impact of Domestic Abuse on the Workplace

The most common indicator for workplace violence is domestic abuse at home. The term we use to describe this is "domestic spillover." That is, domestic abuse at the home often spills over to the victim's workplace. It is critical for every firm to have an established, effective means by which your employees can report domestic abuse. Employees need to have a portal or reporting mechanism where they can report abuse in which they are the victim or report the abuse of a fellow co-worker. Have you informed your reception, security team, human resources, or legal department about these potential threats? Do you have intervention capable employees to step in and help diffuse conflicts or violence? What are your legal requirements to protect your employees?

Employees need to be trained on how to respond to workplace incidents, violence, and cybersecurity intrusions so they know what to do when an incident occurs. Prior planning and training, and proper incident response can mean the difference between chaos and control, lives lost or saved, and the possible loss of millions of dollars in potential lawsuits and damage to reputation, or not.

Daily news reports detailing incidents of domestic violence are an unfortunate reality across our nation. Recent active shooter events in the workplace, such as the December 2015, San Bernardino, California, incident that killed fourteen and wounded twenty-two—and the April 2018, San Bruno, California, shooting at the YouTube headquarters—remind us that domestic violence often spills over into the workplace, resulting in catastrophic loss of life. Domestic violence can manifest itself as physical violence, or as psychological and emotional abuse. Domestic violence occurs unilaterally across all ethnic, racial, and cultural lines, and there has been no relationship established between domestic violence and educational or economic status. According to FBI crime statistics, one in five women in the United States has been a victim of domestic abuse.

The workplace is frequently one of the places domestic abuse victims feel the safest. They seek refuge and security at work. Unfortunately, it is also where abusers know their victims can routinely be found. The leading cause of death for women in the workplace is homicide, and a current or former partner is often responsible for over 30 percent of these deaths. Given these statistics, it is imperative that the company takes active steps to protect employees, prevent domestic violence spillover into the workplace, and proactively respond to violent offenders who enter the premises.

Develop a Corporate Culture of Safety

Most manufacturing facilities and large workshops do an excellent job of making "safety first" a priority. They often post large signs to remind their employees to "Think Safety" as they count the number of days without a work-related injury. However, many nonmanufacturing firms, such as corporate offices, law firms, and large data processing centers do not feel that safety is a primary issue when in fact it's essential. The safety and well-being of employees needs to become a corporate value regardless in what industry the company operates.

Another hurdle employers have to overcome is that employees who are victims of domestic abuse are frequently reluctant to talk about their situations. The employees may fear the social stigma of victimization or may even feel their abuse is warranted. Policies on workplace violence should be frequently distributed to every employee, which should help in addressing these fears and concerns. These policies must be endorsed and communicated from the top down.

The most important security component in a company is its chief executive offer, or CEO. If the CEO is not committed to a philosophy of security, the entire company is at risk. The head of a firm not only controls the budget and guides the hiring policy, but his or her thinking spreads throughout the company. If the CEO believes in security, other managers will follow—and so will the employees. The company CEO, president, or founder must take an active role in supporting these programs for them to be effective. These program policies need to be effectively conveyed to all employees, at every level, and must encourage workers to come forward when they need help.

Make your company a safe haven for domestic abuse victims. Assure your employees that your firm is there to help and assist in every way possible and let them know that while they are at work, they will be safe. Have counselors on staff or on-call to assist with any cry for help. Ensure the offenders of any domestic violence are positively identified and prevented from entering your workplace. Train your first-line supervisors to recognize the signs of a victim of domestic abuse.

A 2005 study by Swanberg and Logan found that victims of domestic violence were significantly concerned about the reactions of their employers if they disclosed their victimization. The very word "domestic" refers to personal matters, something that occurs at home and should stay at home. This stigma of domestic violence often prevents victims (your employees) from disclosing their situation. Be the exception and develop a healthy work environment that openly discusses domestic violence, as well as its impact on productivity and the safety and security of your other employees.

Anti-violence policies can be used to change workplace culture and create an environment where domestic violence victims are encouraged to notify the appropriate security personnel, human resources, or counseling services. The policies must encourage full disclosure even when the threats may not seem serious. In this regard, it is essential for employees to have consistent and reliable ways to confidentially report threats and concerns about domestic violence. Once these concerns are known, the company's security, safety, and legal personnel will be able to take the necessary steps to secure the workplace. A strong security and safety plan will help minimize the number of domestic violence related incidents in the workplace.

Recognize Pre-Incident Indicators

While there is no single profile of a victim or an offender of domestic violence, there are behaviors that have been shown to frequently precede extreme acts of violence. It is important for the human resources department, security personnel, the receptionist, customer service professionals, and managers to familiarize themselves with the warning signs. By recognizing pre-incident warning signs, you increase the chances to lessen the threat and prevent acts of violence. Some warning signs or behaviors that are recognized as being associated with domestic violence include:

- **Victim tardiness and absenteeism:** Twenty-five percent of the women who claimed that they were in an abusive relationship reported that the abuse has caused them to be late for work on multiple occasions. Employees in abusive relationships lose an average of seven days of work every year due to domestic violence.

- **Victim's inexplicable injuries and frequent reports of accidents:** It is very common for those in abusive relationships to appear at work with black eyes, swollen joints, and other bumps and bruises.

- **Frequent calls and visits to the workplace by the abuser:** Abusive behavior is often an attempt to control the person who is being abused. The offender's frequent visits and calls are to determine with whom the victim talks and visits.

- **Threats:** Threats of violence are intended to direct behavior and an abuser will often use threats of violence to control a relationship. Moreover, it is not uncommon for an abuser to threaten employees who come to the defense of a victim.

According to the American Institute on Domestic Violence (2001), as many as 75 percent of domestic violence victims face harassment from intimate partners while they are at work. In addition, as many as 96 percent experience problems at work due to abuse, 56 percent are late to work, 28 percent leave work early, and 54 percent miss entire days at work. This is certainly a productivity and safety issue that should be handled at the workplace.

No security plan is 100 percent effective or capable of stopping every incident of workplace violence. However, you can introduce a plan that will help mitigate workplace violence and lessen the severity of the acts should they occur. Although recognizing the early warning signs of domestic violence is key, it is not enough on its own to prevent acts of violence. It is essential to respond to the warning signs and to address the issues as they occur.

All supervisors should be trained to initiate counseling sessions with employees as soon as they notice behavior indicating an employee is having trouble. First level supervisors are the eyes and ears of the organization. They have more face-to-face contact with employees than any other level of management, but they need not be alone when dealing with potentially problematic situations. Even when the appropriate intervention has been made, supervisors should not make decisions in a vacuum. Have written policies that dictate notification be made to human resources, security, senior leadership, and the legal department when employees voice concerns regarding safety matters. If threats have been made, it would also be prudent to contact local law enforcement.

Communication Is Key

Policies are most effective when they are widely distributed and clearly communicated to employees. Employees suffering from domestic violence must understand that their employers will help keep them safe, but they must also understand their role in keeping their co-workers safe. Employees must be empowered to believe they are the most important cog in the security plan. Managers need to publicize their workplace violence policies in email reminders, post them in common areas, discuss them with new hires, and bring them to the forefront during board meetings and all-employee conferences.

Equally important, employers should have a written policy for what to do during an active shooter event (ASE) or other violent incident. Specific actions on how to respond during an ASE will be discussed in detail later in this chapter. Companies have an obligation to inform and train their employees on how to properly react to a violent incident. The most important action to take is to move. Get out of the building or the area of the active shooter. If you can't escape, prepare to defend yourself.

It is essential that the general physical security plans of your company convey a safe work environment to your employees. Security measures that can impact the employee's perception of safety and security are: effectively managing your emergency exits and entrances, implementing strict entry procedures and visitor protocols, securing parking lots, and employing CCTV surveillance of the property. Other preventive measures include an effective communication system to notify and inform employees of potential threats, as well as working with local law enforcement to keep them informed of acts of domestic violence, and utilizing the legal department to seek restraining orders if necessary.

Preventing workplace violence requires a group effort. Workplaces are safer when all employees are educated and aware of the signs of domestic violence, and know what steps to take to prevent violent incidents. Employers should ensure that their workplace violence policies are robust and constantly evolving to respond to potential threats. Ultimately, it is the employer's preparation and commitment to protect his employees that creates the power to save lives.

When an employer's actions consistently demonstrate a commitment to safety, there is a dual effect: it limits a violent offender's ability to inflict harm, and it also inspires employees to report their concerns.

How to Empower Your Employees

Companies need to create security awareness in all of their employees. The difficulty is doing this without creating paranoia, frightening them with PowerPoint presentations, or boring them to the extent they stop caring about security! Empowering your employees, that is, making each of them feel that they are an important part in the security plan, is the key to success. Everyday safety needs to be communicated from the CEO down to the receptionist and custodial services, and it requires the participation of every employee.

How do you do this? How do you **empower your employees**?

Explain to your employees that they need to be able to save themselves in an emergency situation. Help them develop their own plan for self-protection! Drill them on where to go and how to get there. Talk to them about using improvised weapons such as pens, scissors, box cutters, hammers, screwdrivers, fire extinguishers, and chairs to fend off an attacker. Think of this in terms of an airline safety brief. Give them an "action plan," but leave enough room for personal improvisation to thwart the unexpected actions of the offender.

Reward participation in your security awareness and reporting programs. Even if you can get only one out of ten people to go along, you'll have increased your security and intelligence team by 10 percent. Develop innovative and fun ways to engage your employees to "think security." I recommend developing a game that has an immediate reward for the winner. For example, I tell my corporate clients to play the Purple Unicorn game. Take a regular-sized business envelope and cover it with stickers of unicorns (finding stickers of purple unicorns is not as difficult as you may think!). Then instruct the chief security officer (CSO) to hide the envelope on the same day, every week. You can call it "Security Wednesday" or "Find the Unicorn Friday" or name the unicorn "Thelma" and call it "Thelma Thursday"—it doesn't matter. The point is to get your employees to think about security awareness, if not every day, at least one day a week.

The CSO hides the unicorn-bedazzled envelope by taping it to the inside of a fire hose panel or on the bottom of a AED (automated external defibrillator) box or the back of the door to a stairwell—anywhere that might help your employees think about safety and security. You can even hide it in plain sight, like in the lobby of your firm where most people operate in "Code White" and do not pay attention to their environment.

Send out an email every Monday morning (or the day of your choice) to "All Employees" titled "Find Me for Money." Include a photo of the envelope and tell them the first person that responds to the email with the location of the unicorn envelope receives a $25 gift certificate to Home Depot, or iTunes, or a local restaurant. In a follow-up email, identify the winner and take a photo of them holding the envelope and the gift certificate. Include a reminder for everyone to always think about safety and security and to report any suspicious behavior or incidents. It's amazing how many employees will end up looking for the envelope while developing their situational awareness and security mindset without consciously knowing they're doing it.

Giving away a $25 gift card once a week is an inexpensive way to increase the security awareness of the employees. For as little as $100 a month, you can dramatically increase the overall protective attitude and safety awareness of your organization.

Not only that, this program will also help develop a friendly and open relationship between the CSO and your company's employees—something that is good for intelligence collection and security awareness.

Another easy way to empower and encourage your employees in regards to security matters is to provide weekly safety tips to all employees via your firm's email system. Examples could include:

- If a robber asks for your wallet or purse—do NOT hand it to them. Throw it toward them, but far enough away that he has to move. He is more interested in your money than in you. When he goes to pick it up—RUN! It's very difficult to hit a moving target with a handgun.

- If you are ever thrown into the trunk of a car, kick out the back tail lights and stick your arm out the hole and start waving like crazy. The driver won't see you, but everybody else will. This tip has saved lives!

- Always keep a tactical flashlight on you and use it at nighttime. Having a light allows you to see better in the darkness, but it can also act as a deterrent for would-be criminals. In today's society, usually it is only police officers that routinely use flashlights. So, if you're seen shining your light as you walk to your car, the bad guys will probably think you're a cop. If worst comes to worst, you can use the tactical flashlight as a defensive tool by blinding your would-be attacker with the bright beam or hitting him with the beveled edge.

- The 911 Emergency Call System is less effective from your mobile phone than it is from the phone on your desk. If you have to dial 911, use a landline whenever possible so the dispatcher can trace your physical location instead of the cell phone tower relaying your call.

These simple safety tips will keep your employees thinking about safety often. You are essentially drafting all of your employees into your security department by making everyone feel that they are a part of the security plan. Let all employees know that they're not alone because workplace violence is a "we problem," and "we need to deal with it as a company."

Empowering your employees with their own sense of preparedness allows them to play an active role in their own security and that of your business. Then if they see something abnormal, they already have the contact email and phone number.

Your Return on Investment in Physical Security

Corporate security, while no different from other business functions, can be more complex to evaluate your return on investment or ROI. At the end of the day, corporate security officers (CSOs) need to demonstrate how their actions and activities add value to the company, just like any other department or division. Across the globe, CSOs are under intense pressure to justify what they do and how much they spend. Business operations are coming under increased scrutiny from the business owners, shareholders, and outside auditors. As a result, CSOs find themselves in the position of needing to make a strong case for their budgets and activities.

Identifying the return on investment on security is a challenging task. Security is an investment that pays for itself in cost savings and cost avoidance, not in generating a return. Physical security is about loss prevention and is calculated via tangibles like time and money, as well as intangibles like employee safety, corporate reputation, and competitive advantage.

During my twenty-year career in the FBI, I was often asked to comment on security in the corporate environment. Today my firm does a lot of security consulting and risk management for companies who are forward thinking and security conscious. These firms want to develop a strategic security plan before they have a serious critical or violent incident. I have seen CSOs use poorly conceived corporate security platform to try to manage a variety of crisis situations, from terrorism to cyber threats, which rapidly spin out of control. Not having a detailed security and crisis management plan, which is communicated and practiced often, can quickly prove disastrous in the event of a critical incident. Security matters, in the face of rapidly unfolding events, should provide the CSO with an opportunity to demonstrate the value and importance of his corporate security plan. While the core mission of corporate security is to develop plans that are both proactive and responsive, the goal remains to mitigate risks to physical safety and to ensure the continuity of operations during a crisis.

In the world of physical security, protection of the company's employees, its assets, and its reputation is paramount. Consider the 2016 tragic bombings in Brussels, Belgium, in which three coordinated suicide attacks occurred. Two attacks occurred at the Brussels Airport, and one at the Maalbeek metro station in the city center. Thirty-two people were killed and over three hundred more were injured.

By monitoring social media, many companies were able to quickly reach out to their employees, and notify them if they were in route, to return to their homes. By using mass media notification messaging, these companies were able to tell their employees who were in the building to shelter-in-place. Throughout the day, the CSO shared updated information in real time to keep their employees informed and most importantly, safe!

These firms obviously had well-written and well-rehearsed Crisis Management Plans and had invested in security for their company and their employees. What is the return on investment if only one employee's life was saved? What is the ROI for minimizing the effect and disruption to business as it relates to this particular terror attack?

In addition to dealing with possible loss of life, firms that were not prepared had to deal with issues relating to business continuity, securing assets and property, securing supply lines, ensuring employee safety, and other duty of care matters. Without an immediate and decisive response, critical business processes like the chain of supply, can be severely compromised. Having a well-trained, active security team allows firms to respond more quickly and efficiently, saving the company untold millions of dollars—that is a good return on investment!

Developing the Survival Mindset

As detailed in the first chapter, developing a survival mindset is critical to survive any crisis situation. Everyone understands the inherent threat of an active shooter. Unfortunately a lot of organizations are reluctant to take steps to mitigate this threat because they may feel the training is too expensive or they're fearful of scaring their employees. They rationalize that "it'll never happen to me" or "if I recognize it as a possible threat, then I am obligated to address it." Instead, business leaders of all levels should understand and actively communicate the importance of preparing for the worst, while training for success. Developing the survival mindset is the first step to surviving a critical incident.

Keeping It Simple

Response to a critical incident never has a one-size-fits-all solution. The right response depends on dozens of variables, including the size of the building, the number of victims, the number of predators, the police response time, the number of exit points, and a host of other factors. While different threats do warrant varying responses, too many procedures can confuse and cripple an organization during a high-stress scenario, which prevents the necessary response.

All active shooter response plans should be built upon one simple principle—**get out**!

Once you have determined that there is an active shooter at your location, make every attempt to get out of the building and away from the threat. Run! Move! Create Distance! Get Out!

Hiding does NOT work! By hiding you are only making yourself and easy target for the predator. The average distance between an active shooter and his victim is less than two feet. The only exception to not running away and creating distance between you and the shooter is if the shooter is between you and the only way out. In that case, barricade yourself in a room—lock the door, prevent the shooter from gaining access to where you are located, and then look for improvised weapons to attack the shooter should he gain access. Remember, improvised weapons can be a fire extinguisher, a pen (preferably a tactical pen), scissors, a broken broom stick, a leg from a chair, or anything else that can be used to defend yourself.

Locking Mechanisms

Employers and organizations need to equip their buildings with a locking system that allows the employees to lock the doors quickly and easily, especially when they are under duress. The ability to quickly secure the door using gross motor skills (remember fine motor skills diminish significantly under stress) is essential to surviving an active shooter event. The ability to quickly deny the shooter access to rooms or areas is the second most important tactic employers can implement after designating an exit strategy.

Employers should also invest in mechanical doorstops, hinge sleeves, or throw bolts that can be used to quickly lock the door. There are numerous types on the market that are very effective and easy to use. Examples include: The Sleeve, The Guardian, Bolo Stick, Night Lock, and many others. Companies and organizations need to determine which mechanism fits their needs best, and then invest in the installation of a door locking system throughout their structure or office areas.

Proactive Response Plans

As a result of the number of active shooter events (ASE), there is a movement in the insurance industry for companies to have an **Active Shooter Plan of Action**. Unfortunately, increased exposure to violence in the workplace is the new normal. An effective response plan doesn't begin when the incident occurs, but long before in the form or training and preparation. People respond well under stress only to the extent to which they have been trained. Effective training is critical to surviving a violent, active shooter event. Also, training employees how to identify and communicate possible high-risk indicators such as signs of growing anger, domestic abuse, depression, or erratic behavior can be effective in identifying a potential active shooter before he or she takes violent action. Remember: Knowledge increases confidence, confidence increases decisiveness, and *it is decisive action in a critical incident that saves lives.*

As with most things, communication is key.

A plan of action based on fundamentals will still fail without clear communication before, during, and after a critical incident. What is said and how you say it plays an important role in the action plan. Be sure the language you use to communicate the event is clear and concise. The plan should include the **avoid, deny, defend** or ADD moniker.

- **AVOID** the shooter at all costs. If you know the shooter's location, create as much distance from the shooter as possible. Get off the X; Leave; Run; Get Out!

- **DENY** the shooter access to your location if you are unable to create distance. Lock the door; secure it with belts, neckties, tables, chairs, anything to prevent the shooter from gaining access to your location.
- **DEFEND** yourself should the shooter gain access to your space. Use any improvised weapon you can find and, if need be, defeat the shooter using your hands and your survival mindset. If you are with others, devise a plan to attack the shooter should he enter your space. Attack the shooter's vulnerable areas: his eyes, throat, knees, and groin.

Communication during a critical incident should not be limited to employees. It should include all customers and visitors. How a company communicates during an active threat incident can play a vital role in minimizing the harm as a result of panic. I recommend not using code words to communicate the presence of an active shooter. Use plain English to notify everyone in the building of the threat to allow for employees, customers, or visitors to take decisive action.

Every active threat situation will unfold differently. External factors such as the building size, number of entry/exit points, windows, number of employees, the floorplan, the locking mechanisms on the doors, and other variables result in an unpredictable outcome—no two active shooter events are the same. By being proactive, companies can be prepared for and respond to an active threat. Through the empowerment of its most valuable assets—its people—companies can mitigate the active shooter risk.

Good Security Is Good Customer Service

Every business should have a small team of trained personnel who can act as the **Intervention Capable Response Team**. In other words, someone who can approach a suspicious person and make contact, ask a few simple questions and ascertain whether that person poses a threat.

Someone trained in basic human nature and nonverbal communications can be an effective intelligence gatherer and deterrent against those with evil intent. Here is how it works—you have a small team of individuals who are looking for those visitors or guests that appear to be anomalies in your environment, someone who does not fit the norm or seems overly nervous or uncomfortable. If the receptionist, the security guard watching the CCTV cameras, or a trained employee observes a visitor who seems to be agitated or nervous, the Intervention Capable Response person is notified and he will greet the visitor, shake his hand, and welcome the individual to the business.

By doing this, the guest who is probably there for valid business reasons, looks at the introduction as great customer service. He will leave later that day and tell his friends how welcomed he felt when he entered your business. In essence, what your Intervention Capable Team is really doing is determining whether or not the visitor was a potential threat. By shaking their hand, you can determine whether they have sweaty palms—often a sign of nervousness or fear. By welcoming them to your business, you can determine whether they make eye contact with you. Avoiding eye contact is also an indicator of fear or nervousness. By talking to them, you are able to decide if the visitor responds to direct questions, such as

- "Is this your first time here?"
- "How can I help you?"
- "Who are you here to see?"

Based on the visitor's verbal response, eye contact, handshake, and overall demeanor, your Intervention Capable Response employee is able to make an informed decision on whether this person poses a threat to your building and your employees. If they are there for legitimate business, the intervention comes across as great customer service. If they are there with ill intent, by approaching, the Intervention Team may be able to dissuade them from action by upsetting their OODA loop decision process, by publically acknowledging them as a potential threat, or by physical intervention if appropriate.

Remember: The OODA loop, "Observe, Orient, Decide, Act" is the decision-making process we all utilize many times a day.

Physical Security of Your Building

Check the physical security of your building from the outside looking in. Then, construct concentric rings of defense so if the outer ring is compromised, an inner security ring will contain the threat. These outer, middle, and inner security rings should include physical barriers such as vehicle stops, fencing, and access card readers. Other deterrents such as lighting, cameras, motion sensors, and behavior barriers such as sign-in/sign-out procedures, routines, and employee awareness all enhance the security posture.

Start with little things that tell your employees that safety and security is the new normal. Insist that the handwriting on all sign-in and sign-out forms is legible and conduct a 100 percent, all-of-the-time ID check. Have your security personnel check that all employees wear their employee credentials around their necks, no exceptions. Require that ID badges be swiped upon both entry and exit to the building—it's the only way to have an accurate count of who's actually in the building at any point in time. If your security team sets and enforces the standard, it will soon become the norm and the expected.

If you routinely have visitors, insist that they sign a logbook (legibly) and show a state issued identification, such as a driver's license. Your security or receptionist should call to confirm the visitor's appointment prior to access into the employee area. The visitor should then be provided with a visitor badge, always escorted within the building and required to sign out before leaving.

Be sure to do routine checks on your HVAC systems (heating, ventilation, and air-conditioning). Look for signs of tampering and ease of access. Today's terrorists are sophisticated and have the skill set to use biological, chemical, or radiological agents that can be dispersed via your HVAC systems.

Be sure the building has crash-proof barriers to prevent someone from driving a large truck into the front lobby. Specialized engineers and architects can design or retrofit buildings to make them bombproof and bulletproof.

As with securing your home, check the perimeter to see if it has blind spots where terrorists or intruders could easily hide. Fencing, security gates, access points, delivery areas, and landscaping should all be a part of your security perimeter defense. Keep shrubs and bushes trimmed low and away from the building's exterior. Be sure to keep a close eye on delivery zones and parking garages, as these are prime areas where terrorists and those with ill intent will attempt to enter your building.

You don't let strangers into your home, so don't let strangers into your business. Don't assume outside contractors have been vetted or have had a background check. Check their credentials and their identification closely before you allow them access. Implementing security turnstiles with an ID badge is a very effective form of physical security, but people still piggyback every day. We are too gracious and want to be thought of as polite. This is where good communication is essential to educate your employees that they need to be an enforcer of security procedures. For example, tell your employees if they do not badge in and out every day, after three violations, you are going to have a discussion with them and their supervisor to discuss behavior issues and not following company guidelines. This is certainly a paradigm shift in the company culture, but it must be done to ensure compliance which improves security.

When starting new construction of an office building, consider designing and installing "safe rooms" or "hardened rooms" for your employees to use in the event of a critical situation such as an active shooter event, or even severe weather. These could be equipped with blast doors, filtered ventilation system, emergency lighting, separate telephone lines, both TV and radio reception, and a supply of food and water.

Dealing with Improvised Explosive Devices

The threat of explosive devices, or Improvised Explosive Devices, more commonly referred to as IEDs, being used in an active shooter event is nothing new. The two Columbine High School shooters who murdered twelve students and one teacher in 1999 had close to one hundred explosive devises, from small hand-thrown IEDs to a large vehicle-borne device. Explosive devices have been used in numerous other incidents.

Both first responders and civilians must be prepared to find these types of devices while training and in real-world incidents. The standard "bomb threat" training currently in place will do little to defend individuals against an adversary who is determined to kill as many people as possible.

The first rule of thumb when dealing with explosives is: "If you can see the device (bomb), it can hurt you." Creating distance and angles from the device is your best and first course of action. If you come across an explosive device such as a pipe bomb, or a suspicious backpack placed in a hallway or in the lobby of your office building, quickly run away and then break off at a ninety-degree angle away from the device.

The effects of an explosion are dependent on the size and explosive-weight of the device. Once the explosion occurs, the shock wave will travel the path of least resistance, much like water would flow after a dam break. The shock wave can be lethal and you need to create as much distance, air gaps, and angles between you and the shock wave as possible. Linear areas such as hallways or enclosed rooms are especially dangerous areas to be in when an explosion occurs.

The Three Rules for Improvised Explosive Devices

Rule #1: NEVER TOUCH THE DEVICE. This includes the box, bag, backpack, or car that houses the device.

Rule #2: CREATE DISTANCE, ANGLES, AND AIR GAPS between you and the device. Remember, if you can see the device, it can hurt you!

Rule #3: LET OTHERS KNOW. Communicate to everyone in the area that a bomb has been located. Evacuate the area and continue to communicate the presence, location and description of the device.

In an office environment, keep an eye out for unattended or unfamiliar bags or backpacks. Employees should be trained to be alert for briefcases, luggage, handbags, or backpacks left unattended in the lobby or near the entrances to your building. Pay particular attention if you see someone gingerly placing an object on the ground, rather than just dropping it. Finally, flying glass is deadly in an explosion. Have your building's windows checked and decide if the installation of anti-shatter film is appropriate.

Physical Security versus Cyber Security—Insider Threats!

Not a day goes by without some discussion, news article, or update on the newest cybersecurity application. Cybersecurity gets a lot of attention, as it should, yet physical security and investigations are still a key element in enterprise security, particularly when it comes to "insider threats." We all understand the severity of data breaches and as a result boards of directors, shareholders, and chief security officers devote a significant amount of time and resources mitigating these threats.

The reason cybersecurity gets so much attention is because of the impact on stock prices a data breach can have on an institution. Insider threat is equally as troublesome if one of your own people does something that catches the media's attention. Bottom line, bad publicity is bad for the company whether it's cyber related or people related.

Employee Screening

Most companies do pre-employment screening; but that is a snapshot in time. I recommend to my clients to continually monitor employees on an ongoing basis. There are a number of services available that will notify the company if an employee is arrested, has a lien placed on their property, declared bankruptcy, or is involved in domestic violence. None of these by themselves are necessarily grounds for dismissal; but they might be "pre-incident indicators" that the employee is under stress, or may need some outside counseling or assistance.

That information can also be extremely valuable in an investigation that may have already been started. It might give an investigator some insight to the totality of the circumstances and be used to construct an interview strategy should the investigation require it.

Continuous monitoring via physical security and IT security is critical in addressing threats to the company posed by disgruntled employees. Companies should take the approach where they communicate to their employees that misbehavior hurts not only themselves, but also their co-workers and their employer.

The importance of training your employees, particularly those who travel overseas or have access to the most sensitive, proprietary information, cannot be overestimated. Train your employees to recognize techniques and tradecraft skills used by foreign government or hostile corporate competitors. These techniques include anything from soft personal introductions, often at trade shows or conferences, to the "honeypot," where a member of the opposite sex is introduced to the employee to entice them into a compromising situation in which blackmail is then used to get the employee to betray the company.

Both law enforcement (FBI and Department of Homeland Security) and the intelligence community are partners with US-based corporations in efforts to defend industry against tradecraft perpetrated by foreign governments and bad actors. I tell all my clients to develop a relationship with the USG (US government), particularly at our embassies, if the firm conducts business overseas.

Tracking and monitoring online activity by your employees is essential in protecting your firm from insider threats. Suspicious online activity, to include irregular information loading or downloading of emails with attachments, is a key indicator in identifying possible insider threats. There are a number of tools available to examine and track online activity and to recognize when there is a deviation from the norm. Much like looking for the anomalies in each environment (see chapter 2 – Situational Awareness) to maintain your situational awareness, tracking anomalies on your company's IT system will also help in identifying that threat from within.

One aspect of security for business leaders that is often ignored or not emphasized is the cybersecurity for their CEO.

It's a gap I've seen in a lot of corporate training I have conducted. Although here in the United States we do not use our intelligence agencies to steal secrets from visiting business executives to advance our commercial interests, other countries most certainly do. Cybersecurity is not just about keeping your cellphone on your person; it's reasonable to believe when traveling overseas, foreign intelligence agents in that country will gain access to your CEO's hotel room and image the laptop left behind while your CEO is enjoying dinner.

It's important to remember a strong security culture results in reduced risk!

We're from the Government and We're Here to Help!

The Department of Homeland Security recently (2018) unveiled its new National Risk Management Center (NRMC), which coordinates efforts to protect US critical infrastructure. The NRMC creates a cross-cutting risk management approach across the federal government and private sector partners through three lines of effort:

- Identifying and prioritizing strategic risks to national critical functions
- Integrating government and industry activities on the development of risk management strategies
- Synchronizing operational risk management activities across industry and government

The Center works closely with the National Cybersecurity and Communications Integration Center (NCCIC), which remains the DHS's central hub for cyber operations. The NMRC runs simulations, tests, and cross-sector exercises, and it serves as a sort of "911" resource for local, state, federal and private organizations in cybersecurity crisis.

Utilizing current infrastructure to help protect your firm is common sense—use government assets if they meet your security needs.

Providing Security for Executives

There are a number of CEOs and other high-net-worth individuals who travel overseas, often to very dangerous places: Central America, Southeast Asia, the Middle East, and Africa just to name a few. Unfortunately it's not unusual for these powerful men of industry and finance to travel without a proper threat assessment, without a crisis action plan or kidnap-for-ransom insurance. In other words, they travel without an accurate "ground truth." These people are at an even greater risk than the average tourist due to their positions, their crucial knowledge concerning their businesses, or their net worth; yet, they often travel as if they were going to Disney World.

A proactive chief security officer (CSO) recognizes the risks of traveling overseas and relays these potential dangers to the CEO. The CSO should provide suggestions to help lessen the known threats and ensure his CEO has the proper level of security coverage in country—based on a thorough threat assessment. The chief security officer should provide the CEO with a detailed security and safety plan, which includes the name, photo, and contact information for a vetted and trained driver, a secure hotel with the name and contact information of the concierge, points of contact at every location to be visited, a means to have immediate communications with the CEO, a communications plan (regular check-in times), a mechanism to track their location, a detailed itinerary, an evacuation plan in the event of a medical emergency or civil unrest, and a Crisis Management Plan in the event the CEO is kidnapped or goes missing.

Hire a seasoned, qualified security professional as CSO. Employing a highly qualified and trained CSO means more than just hiring a competent retired police officer. A true security professional that is well versed in counter-terrorism, physical security and cybersecurity usually comes from government agencies such as the FBI, CIA, or USSS. Be sure your CSO is connected with the local FBI office and attends its Citizen Academy. Have your CSO join the local ASIS chapter (ASIS is the world's largest membership organization for security management professionals), the FBI's InfraGard program (InfraGard is a nonprofit organization serving as a public-private partnership between US-based businesses and the FBI), and any other security organizations or associations that promote communication of ideas and intelligence. (Note: InfraGard provides a means for seamless public-private collaboration with the US government that provides an exchange of information relevant to the protection of our nation's critical infrastructure).

A proactive, alert chief security officer who is not afraid to think outside the box will also provide hands-on-training for all employees, including any senior management who travels overseas. This training would include situational awareness, tactics and techniques to avoid a kidnapping, how to escape from inside a locked trunk of a vehicle, how to escape from handcuffs (it's a lot easier than you think), duct tape, rope, or flex-ties; and how to disarm someone pointing a gun in your face. Teaching "tradecraft" skills to senior executives will be fun, yet arm them with skills that could potentially save their lives.

If your CSO is not providing a pre-travel intelligence and threat briefing prior to C-suite executives traveling overseas, or if your company or firm is too small to have a fully staffed corporate security office and you are not taking the appropriate pre-travel measures for yourself, then you are traveling with the hope that nothing bad will happen—that is just foolish.

For smaller firms, look to outside experts and bring them in, under contract, to train your employees in tradecraft skills.

Ask them if they have overseas contacts in law enforcement or intelligence agencies and have them provide ground truth and a written Risk and Vulnerability Assessment. A lot of information can be gleaned by looking at the US State Departments Travel Advisory website and other open source data bases.

In a previous chapter I told you how the one of biggest risk to any traveler in a foreign country is getting into a taxicab, and that most robberies, abductions, and violent crime occur in or near a vehicle. Therefore, it is essential that pre-travel security plans be prepared by the CSO, using only trusted and vetted suppliers of drivers and vehicles. Relying on taxis and ride-share services has led to many kidnappings, violent assaults, and the deaths of executives traveling throughout the world.

The CSO must be a leader who is able to effectively communicate with the senior executives to make sure they understand the logic behind the security measures being proposed. It also means solid training and briefings for every traveler in the firm. It will require an adaptive, agile, and highly trained Executive Protection Team, a robust protective intelligence program, and liaison contacts across the globe. These take time, money, manpower, regular training, and a commitment to improving every day. The return on investment will be readily apparent in the event of an actual crisis situation. It also ensures a long-lasting and sustainable corporate security department, one that is appreciated and funded by the board and other key shareholders.

Information collection and dissemination is a critical part of an effective security program. It is not enough to just collect information and share it within the security department; this relevant and actionable intelligence has to be communicated to your C-suite executives and other business travelers. This will make your firm more dependable by enabling its executive travelers to operate safely in challenging environments.

Why Executive Protection for the CEO?

I am often asked why corporations establish executive protection programs for their CEOs and other employees. The question is fair enough, since corporate executive protection is a relatively new phenomenon for many companies, can be very expensive, and by its very nature not something that people outside the boardroom discuss much in public.

But the more I think about an answer, the more I am convinced that the question should be turned on its head. A better question is, Why wouldn't corporations establish executive protection programs for their CEOs and other C-level employees?

I had the distinct honor of being the FBI's Hostage Rescue Team (HRT) Dignitary Protection Program Manager during the last three years of my time on the Team. As a result I was sent to both a United States Secret Service (USSS) school and a United States Diplomatic Security Service (DSS) School for Dignitary Protection, or more commonly called "Executive Protection" (EP). These schools provided me with the knowledge, tactics, and procedures to then teach the new HRT operators how to conduct executive protection operations. It is a very difficult skill set to master. In fact, an entire federal agency was established just to conduct executive protection operations—the United States Secret Service—and they are the best in the world at what they do!

Corporate executive protection is a relatively new discipline in the corporate world. As a result, there are a lot of misconceptions and misinformation on corporate EP programs. I have seen many EP teams, both domestically and internationally, who truly have no idea how to conduct a personal protection detail. In an EP operation, the devil is definitely in the details. That is to say, there are a lot of vulnerabilities to consider and mitigation of risks, which have to be planned for. There are arrivals and departures, protection while in transit and at the various locations, and with the countless people with whom your principal will be meeting. Every EP program is based on one philosophy—keep the principal safe! In the EP world, the word "safe" is defined as being protected from danger, risk, injury, threats, and embarrassment. Yes, the principal's reputation must also be secured.

Executive Protection—It's about Productivity

Although it is impossible to be completely safe at all times, a good EP team will do everything they can to alleviate risks. Often this will include reducing the principal's exposure to dangers at work, home, and while traveling. A good EP program will increase the productivity of the principal by allowing him to stay focused on his work no matter where that work takes him. This productivity supports the return on investment on the security program and it keeps the board members happy knowing their CEO is safe and out of harm's way. A good EP program increases the CEO's mobility and their effectiveness. It's not just safety and security; it's taking care of personal needs before he even arrives, like checking into the hotel, having cars and trained drivers at the ready, and knowing the fastest and safest routes to various meeting locations.

It is always interesting to me when I do security assessments for Fortune 500 companies to see how many have never considered formulating a corporate EP strategy. A lot of the companies with whom I have contracts, have a "reactive security strategy," employing a "wait-and-see" plan that only changes when circumstances demands it.

There is a reason the CEO has a personal assistant, travels by company jet or in business class, and doesn't have to write up the minutes of every meeting he attends: productivity. Executive protection, in addition to keeping the CEO safe, also enables higher productivity by making travel and everyday logistics run as smoothly as possible. Secure travel eliminates waiting for cabs or at the car rental counter. Unlike a ride with a chatty (and often un-vetted and potentially dangerous) hired driver, it also minimizes interruptions, turns travel time into work time, and lets high-paid C-level executives attend more meetings, in more places, in less time, thereby being more productive.

Considering that 85 percent of attacks on protectees (those being protected) have happened in or around a vehicle, having a well-trained security driver is critical to a successful executive protection program. If your CEO is driving himself to and from work each day, he is wasting valuable time where he could be productive, making calls, fine-tuning his daily schedule, etc. A well-trained driver is essential to ensure the principal is able to get from Point A to Point B safely and timely. They are trained to recognize potential threats on the road and to maneuver safely around them. Untrained drivers can end up costing the company time, money, and potential public relations nightmares.

As with any security plan, a good corporate EP program is grounded in the company's corporate culture and the personal preferences of those being protected. Without this backing and support, the program will not be effective. Also, corporate EP programs should be designed for all employees. After all, safety applies to everyone in the corporation, from the CEO to the IT service technician traveling to crime-ridden Honduras. Providing a security team for a mid-level employee traveling to a dangerous location will buy immense loyalty and dedication from the rest of the employees. Having the employees know, without a shadow of a doubt, that the company has their safety as its prime objective will result in huge dividends when it comes to employee loyalty and work productivity.

Given the circumstances, threat assessment, risk analysis, prominence, popularity, vulnerabilities, the lifestyle of their

CEO and innumerable other factors, many corporate boards find it prudent and reasonable to a have a high standard of executive protection for their CEO. Everything else being equal, if one corporation's CEO is more productive and safer than another's, that's a competitive advantage. What board wouldn't want its chief executive to be safer and more productive?

Starting an Executive Protection Program? Ask a Lot of Questions!

Whether you are starting an EP program or just refining your current program, you need to conduct a thorough threat assessment and risk analysis. You need to identify the individuals who are critical to your organization, and conduct a similar assessment on their lives—their very personal lives.

Creating a "protectee"or "principal profile" requires the chief security officer to delve deeply into the personal life of his CEO. This cannot be done without the full cooperation of the principal. You need to know his habits, where he likes to visit, his favorite eateries, details about his home, car, and family; every aspect of his life needs to be viewed with a critical eye looking for vulnerabilities, habits, and potential threats.

Based on what the CSO learns, he will be able to identify security measures needed to keep the principal safe. Once these measures have been identified, it's up to the CSO to justify to the board why the company needs these procedures, equipment, cameras, personnel, and training and then have it budgeted. Security is cheap! Good security is not! A good executive protection team can cost well over half a million dollars per year.

It's important to recognize that vulnerabilities, threats, and risks change over the course of time. A good EP team leader understands this and alters his strategic security plan accordingly. A principal may get dozens of threatening emails a week without the threat level increasing. However, if a threatening letter is delivered to his mailbox or front door, that indicates someone has done their research and has taken great pains to deliver that threat in person. With that scenario, the threat level just got significantly higher.

Starting an Executive Protection Program? Size Doesn't Matter!

The term "Personal Protection Officer" or "Executive Protection Professional" should tell you all you need to know about the evolution of executive security details. Bearded, tattooed, chest-thumping, bro-bumping, no-neck guys wearing the latest Crye Precision combat pants are fine if you want to hit a dance club with a posse; but they are not effective for executive protection. An effective EP program is based on knowledge, intelligence, training, research, and preparation—not on muscle mass.

The difference between a bodyguard and a Personal Protection Officer (PPO) is a bodyguard specializes in muscles and has a gun; a PPO is better prepared to identify a threat before it materializes. He also has a gun, but he knows his brain is his most important and lethal weapon. Keep in mind, in the storied history of the United States Secret Service, their Special Agents have *never* fired a shot conducting protective operations! They know their first priority is to "*cover and evacuate*" their Principal, not to engage in a gun battle. The primary selection criteria for a Secret Service Agent are intelligence, attention to details, and the ability to think under stress. These attributes enable them to reduce the vulnerabilities of their Protectee. As a result of this risk mitigation, no Secret Service Agent has ever had to fire his weapon while protecting the President of the United States.

The perfect PPO is highly intelligent and articulate. He is trained in defensive tactics, firearms skills, defensive driving, and emergency medical training, and he has the ability to defend the principal against an attack. The PPO needs to be able to mimic the principal in professional dress and demeanor, while also blending into the environment. One of the goals of every EP team leader is to minimize the impact of a security detail on the protectee's daily life. Remember, the skills necessary to do EP can be learned; professionalism, discretion, integrity, and dedication are ingrained and more difficult to find. Look for those characteristics long before you look for brawn and muscle mass.

Starting an Executive Protection Program? Customer Service Is Key!

I do a lot of executive protection training, some for newly licensed PPOs and some for well-established EP teams assigned to a principal. I tell them all the same thing: "Ninety-nine point nine percent of your problems or issues in EP can be solved with a firm handshake and a smile." I truly believe this. If a PPO is drawing his weapon while his team leader is covering and evacuating the principal, the EP team has most probably made a mistake. The team missed something it should have seen or anticipated. The chances of a PPO ever being in a gunfight on a protection operation are very slim. In fact, the job of a PPO can (and should) be quite uneventful. It is all the prior planning and the advance work, that will be the biggest factor in keeping the principal and the EP team safe.

Having good organizational abilities, research skills, and good intelligence collection will prevent most problems facing an EP operation. One of the greatest attributes you provide to your principal is the ability to eliminate many of the usual, but petty, travel annoyances. When your principal has last-minute changes to his or her travel plans (and they always do), the professional Personal Protection Officer needs to be in a position to mitigate the new risks, rather than simply respond to them.

Advance work is the key to most successful (i.e. uneventful) executive protection operations. Anticipating the movement, the needs, the desires, and the requirements of your principal is vital to an EP operation's success. Understanding that usually the number one threat to any EP operation is a medical emergency, not an attempted kidnapping, will make the advance work much easier resulting in a better prepared EP team.

Good advance work takes time. It could require two weeks to plan a five-day overseas trip for your principal. It's also an opportunity for the EP team to be viewed as more of a perk than a pain for the principal. The protection professional is both the customer service representative and the concierge for the CEO. The PPO's goal in conducting the advance is to do all the grunt work ahead of the arrival to ensure his principal's visit is seamless and safe. Executives concerned that security will be cumbersome can learn how the organizational prowess of their EP team can make everything run more smoothly.

Starting an Executive Protection Program? Hire a Skilled Investigator!

It is the job of the Executive Protection team to ensure the safety of the principal and of his organization's reputation. A large part of that includes a strong "Protective Intelligence" program that conducts thorough and continual threat assessments. Good threat assessments are done by a skilled investigator.

A good protective intelligence program will identify potential threats, bad actors, security risks, vulnerabilities, and the best vehicle routes, as well as aid in the development of emergency response procedures, luggage control, food preparation, and other details which help ensure your CEO's physical safety and the company's brand and reputation.

I have found a thorough protective intelligence program is best done by an experienced investigator with excellent analytical skills in order to obtain information from multiple independent sources, to include open source information.

Open source intelligence, known as OSINT, is a critical and essential tool to be used in developing your protective intelligence for your principal. The skill to be able to obtain and analyze social media platforms, public records, podcasts, blogs, and news articles, which can provide a wealth of information and intelligence. Looking at social media posts and status updates of persons or groups known to have threatened your principal can help you in planning your routes, which hotel to stay at, and where to eat, and help determine if a legitimate threats exists.

The collection of OSINT should not stop with the pre-planning of the travel or the completion of the threat assessment. Continual, real-time monitoring of social media and other open source outlets should be done while the principal is traveling to identify developing risks such as severe weather, civil unrest, or pandemic outbreaks.

A skilled investigator will also have developed outstanding interview skills. Being able to talk to strangers, establish rapport, and be able to assess the person's mental state and truthfulness is key to developing your protective intelligence report. As with any skilled investigator, they must be approachable with good "people skills" and able to develop confidential sources and contacts who can be relied upon to continually provide up-to-date, real-time intelligence.

Starting an Executive Protection Program? It's All About Who You Know!

Good information is critical to an effective executive protection program. Your EP team leader needs to have the professionalism, manners, communication skills, and panache to work closely with executive assistants, hotel personnel, airline staff, and event organizers. But that's only part of the information network a protection professional needs. Another critical resource for any EP team is having a contact list full of law enforcement officers and fellow security professionals.

During my global travels with the FBI's Hostage Rescue Team and while assigned to our embassy in Budapest, Hungary, I have collected over a thousand business cards from police officers, intelligence officers, private security professionals, concierges, restaurant managers, limo drivers, other PPOs, and a host of other service providers, knowing that one day I may need their services. I've never thrown away a single card!

This has paid huge dividends in my current private security firm. These contacts provide a wealth of knowledge and can provide information on ground truth, current threats, changing political winds, and other factors that can affect the safety and security of your principal. You never know when a security colleague or former contact may have just traveled to the same location for which you're about to depart and can provide you with up-to-date threat information on your destination. When traveling abroad, or to an unfamiliar city, some of the best information can come from your EP peers who have recently worked in the area.

Starting an Executive Protection Program? Rethink Air Travel!

If your company uses a private jet for executive travel, there are other special considerations that need to be addressed. Many executives avoid commercial carriers now in favor of their private corporate jet, especially after all the security delays that were implemented after 9/11. However, corporations with their own aircraft need to rethink security, especially when traveling overseas. Never rely on foreign airport security to guard your plane while it's parked overnight on the tarmac. Hire your own security force to stand watch overnight. Be sure the caterer delivering the food for your return flight is someone you can trust; or better yet, have the flight crew pick up meals from the hotel for the flight home. Be sure every piece of luggage that is put on the plane is accounted for.

Starting an Executive Protection Program? Don't Forget the Wife and Kids!

The most vulnerable people in the corporation may not be the executives under the protection of a professional executive protection team, but instead, it may be their spouse or children, who are far more accessible and are often left out of security planning. If someone intends to cause harm, and they know that an executive has 24-hour security at the office and when he travels, they will look for an easier target—that target is typically the spouse or children.

Be sure your plan to secure the C-level executives includes his or her family. Consideration should be given to provide a protection team at the residence, provide in-home security systems monitored at the corporate security offices, build in-home safe rooms, provide armored vehicles, or conduct additional training to the family members. Be sure to look at commonsense gaps in your security plan, then make the appropriate modifications.

There is never a more welcomed compliment to a security team than your principal telling you, "I hardly know you guys are even here!"

Don't Be a Static Thinker

All successful businesses know that if they don't change with the times, they're doomed for extinction. Static thinking in the business environment is a recipe for a short-lived business; the same goes for security. It is a mistake to become a static thinker in designing and implementing a strategic security plan. Always look for ways to improve your security—look for the emerging threats, recognize new vulnerabilities as they occur, keep abreast of technological advances, and research the new techniques and procedures of innovative security thinkers to stay ahead of the curve.

Crisis Action Plans, Continuity of Operations Plans, and Contingency Plans are essential for any company that wants to survive in today's more dangerous world. If an emergency incident occurs overseas, police and national emergency medical services are often inadequate, overwhelmed, or nonexistent. There must be a pre-identified and rehearsed service in place to ensure an effective and timely response to an emergency.

There are three components to an effective crisis response:

- Communication – The benchmark is to be able to identify the exact location of all employees and be able to effectively communicate with them within minutes of a critical incident.
- Crisis Management – The design and implementation of a plan that allows the Crisis Management Team to react quickly and efficiently. Ensure they are trained and have conducted multiple exercises in a variety of crisis.
- Emergency Evacuation and Shelter-in-Place Plans – These plans should be short, concise, easily communicated and posted throughout the building in the event of a full or partial evacuation, or an order to shelter-in-place.

Remember, terrorists and predators will select their targets and balance the importance of their act against the security they observe. A tempting target will be skipped if security is deemed too tight. Do not let the cost be a deciding factor when it comes to investing in new security measures, whether it is equipment, training, or manpower. Make your company a hard target—IT WILL SAVE LIVES!

Chapter 8
SPECIAL EVENT SECURITY

I had the privilege of being selected by the Dallas FBI as Special Agent-in-Charge for the security planning and implementation for the 2011 NFL Super Bowl hosted in Dallas, Texas. I was asked to oversee the entire security procedure for this major event. Little did I know to what extent the planning and personnel selection would entail.

The security planning for Super Bowl XLV started on the Monday after Super Bowl XLIV. Over seventy federal, state, and local agencies were involved and had to be coordinated to ensure the safety of over 500,000 spectators. I learned that the Super Bowl is not just a one-day event held on the first Sunday in February. The Super Bowl is a week-long affair filled with parties, press meetings, practices, conventions, and more. Although most stadiums that host the Super Bowl hold under 100,000 spectators, there are four to five NFL affiliated guests, vendors, partiers, and players for every ticketed spectator. Hence, a half million visitors came to Dallas to be a part of NFL history. It was truly a team effort to design the security plan for such an event and it would not have been possible without the professionalism and dedication of the men and women of the Dallas FBI, Arlington Police, Irving Police, Fort Worth Police, Dallas

Police, Texas Department of Public Service, NFL Security, FBI Special Event Management Unit, and many, many others.

Fortunately for us, the NBA World Finals were also held in Dallas just weeks before the Super Bowl. This provided a unique opportunity to see our security plan in action and make any adjustments necessary. I felt extremely blessed to have had that opportunity to iron out some wrinkles, which then enhanced the overall security of Super Bowl XLV.

Since 9/11, the US government has taken the security of large-scale, public events seriously, while spending hundreds of millions of dollars each year on the Super Bowl alone. The event is televised worldwide and has one of the largest television audiences every year. Obviously that makes it a prime target for terrorists, and therefore it is afforded the best security planning available.

However, it is the smaller "special events" that are now being targeted by terrorist and active shooters because they know those smaller events provide a much "softer" target. Nowhere was this more evident than in 2016 at the Bastille Day (French Independence Day) celebration in Nice, France, when a nineteen-ton white cargo truck deliberately drove into the crowd, killing over eighty people; or at the Manchester Arena (UK) during the 2017 Ariana Grande concert when a suicide bomber killed twenty-two young concert goers.

These types of smaller events have historically been ignored by security professionals. Even though they all had the requisite number of police officers on-site, the practices that have been shown to be effective in securing larger scale, public or private, indoor or outdoor, and special events were implemented. Special event security cannot just be a line item or checked box. Security must be foremost in the minds of every event planner and every special event host.

As any special event security manager will tell you, no two events are exactly the same. Special event planning, response, and management are often case-by-case operations, and for venue security leaders, this can mean revising or even rewriting the "playbook" for each event.

Security for special events is like the theater—it's a live performance with a huge cast and a lot of moving pieces. No two performances and no two events are identical. There are a multitude of things that can change without notice, and as in theater, you must be prepared to adjust your role accordingly. It can be different every time, but the bottom line is to ensure a safe and enjoyable event where security is seen as an asset, and not a functional liability or expensive requirement. Guests want to feel safe, they want to see security, but they definitely do not want to be inconvenienced by security.

A Paradigm Shift

Being "good enough" isn't sufficient when it comes to providing security for special events. When large numbers of people gather in a confined area, they become an inviting and easy target for anyone with evil intent. Having the attitude, "It will never happen to me," is not a good security plan. Security cannot be the first line item to be reduced when budget considerations become necessary. A culture shift must occur so event organizers take security seriously.

One of the first changes that need to be implemented is the hiring and training of your security personnel. Large venues, such as sports stadiums, have hundreds of personnel, usually wearing a "Security" windbreaker or polo shirt, to assist in maintaining order and reporting criminal behavior. These security officers are critical to the safety and security of the event. These individuals—along with the parking attendants, ushers, beer vendors, and the popcorn guy—all need to be trained in customer service and security. These people have the most contact with guests (spectators) and will communicate the level of professionalism of your event based on their attire, attitude, and interaction with the guests. These employees are also the eyes and ears for your Security Director; they will see and hear of potential risks long before anyone else.

In today's world, security is complex because the threats are complex. Who would have predicted a deranged man would bring over twenty weapons into his hotel room on the 32nd floor, break two windows of his corner room, and kill 58 concert goers from over 400 yards away? This happened at the Mandalay Bay Hotel in Las Vegas in 2017. This act of cowardice has certainly changed the way concert organizers look at their security plan—as well as it should. Fortunately, most open-air events are not in areas subject to this same type of sniper threat.

Before focusing on the unique risk that the Vegas attack revealed, it is crucial to maintain the fundamentals of layered security for special events. Organizers and their security teams should take this opportunity to assess the primary areas of vulnerability. The focus needs to be on the reasonable steps necessary to reduce these risks. Where is an attack most likely to occur? What is the most likely method of attack? How can we best detect, disrupt and deter a potential attack? These are the questions that need to be answered far in advance of any future event so that risks can be mitigated before they become a reality.

The bottom line is that when planning security for special events, one needs to remember that a good threat analysis and assessment are essential parts in determining where security managers should focus. As horrific as the Las Vegas shooting was, the focus should be on the vulnerabilities, which are related to the event we are currently working to protect.

Layered Security for Special Events

Security at most events has been traditionally handled by local law enforcement or off-duty police officers hired by the event organizers to provided armed security. Most event organizers believe that alerting the local police of the event, and having them present, constitutes a "security plan." The thought behind this is the visual deterrent that uniformed police have on would-be criminals. However, a simple show of force is not sufficient to properly secure an event.

Having police officers on-site is certainly a necessary element in the security plan for every special event. Posting uniformed officers does act as a deterrent for criminal situations that may occur in their line of sight. However, the reaction to a visible security force is similar to a speeding driver who sees a police car and slows down. Once the police car is out of sight, the driver resumes his speeding. Securing a special event, regardless of its size, requires a layered approach that includes law enforcement, private security, technology, counter surveillance, and intelligence collection.

Law Enforcement

The first layer is law enforcement. Every special event needs to have highly visible, uniformed, armed police officers on-site to deter crime, and to assure those attending that security is in place for their protection. If a critical situation does occur, the police are there to respond, conduct crowd control, and assist in securing the crime scene. Uniformed police officers are critical to every Special Event Security Plan.

Private Security

Private security firms need to be contracted early in the planning stages in order to ensure that a well thought out security plan is written, communicated, and implemented. The private security firm is critical in order to collect intelligence and information on possible threats that will be incorporated in a Security Risk Assessment. This written assessment takes place far in advance of the event and is updated continuously until the event has ended.

Private security firms should work closely with event organizers, venue management, vendors and caterers, wait staff, performers, personal protection details, and local police and fire departments to address vulnerabilities and develop the security plan. Each of these components needs to be aware of the security plan, and what to do in the event of a disturbance or attack. The variety of incidents could vary from a missing child to an unattended bag to an active shooter. Private security should also be leveraging their global network of resources and contacts to monitor the current threat level to determine vulnerabilities and risk.

When my firm, Shaffer Security Group, conducts security operations at special events, I like them to blend into the environment, where we can continually collect information and intelligence to share with local police, event organizers, and other team members. By dressing like a guest, my team can get much closer to those who have been identified as suspicious and track their movements while developing a plan to take action should it be warranted.

For special event organizers, it is important that they communicate to all employees and vendors that the private security firm is designated as the Security Director for the event, and it needs to be identified as having complete authority over the security plan and the off-duty, local police, hired as part of that security plan. The police have authority only over criminal acts. This often-tenuous relationship needs a skilled, experienced professional to act as liaison with the local police. The security firm needs to be authorized by the event organizer very early in the planning process so that they can influence the logistics that would impact security.

Unfortunately, most private security firms do not have the much-needed experience to design security plans for special events. Managers and event organizers who are responsible for coordinating special events must assiduously search for experienced private security firms. Ones that are skilled in managing all aspects of the layered approach, and know how to keep everyone informed of changes, developments, and threats, while monitoring their intelligence sources for updated information.

Technology in Security

Advances in technology have certainly had a huge influence on how security operations are conducted and it has never been more evident than in Special Event Security. Technology in security now allows us to monitor social media sights with geo-fencing, and to install perimeter cameras with facial and object recognition capabilities. It also consists of state-of-the-art "shot detection or localization" software, which instantly identifies the location of gunfire and communicates the information on any number of cell phones. There are now air sniffers that can detect the presence of chemical, biological, radiological, and explosive materials.

A Special Event Security Plan gives us the ability to

- Monitor all social media and the dark-net, looking for offensive or threatening content
- Identify individuals through facial recognition on over two thousand databases, or compared against a list of those that have been identified as a threat

- Provide weapon detection via magnetometers, air sniffers, or other available high-end detection systems able to detect certain metal alloys
- Monitor shooter localizations systems, which instantly detects, identifies, and communicates the location of the shooter both indoors and out
- Notify communication networks, which quickly and cost effectively combines information gathering, situational awareness, and secure messaging capabilities

These high-tech security options, when correctly implemented as part of a Special Event Security Plan, could have a huge impact on the safety and security of your event.

Special Event Security Planning and Principles

I could author an entire book just on special event security planning and principles. There is a voluminous amount of information on the subject, and detailed instructions are available from the Department of Homeland Security and others. The concepts are not difficult; however, the implementation of the concepts is very difficult.

In the pre-planning phase, a special event security manager will address a multitude of challenges and principles. The plan must weigh all the security measures that could conceivably be taken, such as street closures, bag searches, and highly visible tactical units, against the event planner's desire to produce an enjoyable, well-attended, and profitable special event. One of his first decisions is to determine the amount of manpower needed for the security workforce. Other challenges include decisions on:

- Access control
- Screening and physical security
- Credentialing

- Transportation
- Intelligence
- Logistics
- Critical infrastructure
- Public health
- Weapons of mass destruction (WMD)
- Crisis management
- Public and media relations
- Training
- Command post operations
- Communications

The best procedure is to plan for the worst-case scenarios—extraordinary crimes, violence by protestors, a possible terrorist attack, and natural disaster—but also be thoroughly prepared to deal with ordinary crimes and incidents, such as fights, drunkenness, a lost child, or small protests.

A security manager must ensure that the event continues safely, but at the same time respect constitutional and human rights, including freedom of speech and assembly. He must establish effective methods of communication and ensure that the rest of his jurisdiction receives essential law enforcement services, regardless of the size or importance of the event. He must not commit all his resources to the special event.

Another layer of security necessary for the security planning of special events is the continual collection of intelligence and information. Security managers must see that appropriate law enforcement and intelligence agencies are informed in advance about events with national or international significance. This is done with physical surveillance, liaison with local businesses, meeting with federal and state law enforcement, and through a global network of contacts that most professional private security firms possess. This will guarantee awareness and assistance in developing a threat assessment. Because threats, vulnerabilities, and situations can change in an instant, it is imperative for the security team to have up-to-date information on any changes.

Too Late, Is Too Late

Frequently, security planning begins far to late in the event planning process. It is important to give your private security team enough time to plan for contingencies and address vulnerabilities. Before the venue is selected, the security manager should be part of the decision-making process in deciding the location, so that a suitable and safe site can be chosen.

I know of one company's nightmare where the firm was hosting a dinner in conjunction with a major sporting event in a large West Coast city. The guest list included many high-profile individuals and celebrities. When the private security firm was contacted, the venue had already been chosen and the event was taking place in a few days.

Unfortunately, the event coordinator did not consider the popularity of the restaurant, and when the VIP guests arrived, it was packed and there was a long line of patrons waiting to get in. Although a private room had been selected, it was on the second floor of the restaurant. There was no plan for how to discreetly get the guests in and out while avoiding delays caused by autograph and selfie seekers. Celebrities risk damaging their reputations if they ignore or refuse their fans' requests, so it created quite a bottleneck. The company was obviously embarrassed and realized that had they brought in an experienced, professional private security consultant during the planning stages, this embarrassment could have been avoided.

Had security been a focus from the start, the recommendation would have been for a different venue that could assure a private, secure access. Choosing a venue is just one aspect that can be positively influenced when security is included in advance of the event. Don't be "too late" in bringing security to the event planning process.

Event planners have a lot to consider, from guest lists to catering, agenda coordination, and so much more. As a result, security concerns can sometimes be left to the last minute. In order to address threats, reduce vulnerabilities, and prevent issues, it takes long-term planning. Having the mentality that says, "It is better to have it and not need it than need it and not have it" will ensure your security plan will be able to address any issue or crisis. In turn, this will provide your event planners and hosts peace of mind. After all, isn't that part of a security professional's job?

Conclusion
MINUTES MATTER

O n September 12, 2001, the day after the 9/11 attacks, British Prime Minister Tony Blair addressed the British Parliament: "The world now knows the full evil and capability of international terrorism, which menaces the whole of the democratic world. The terrorists responsible have no sense of humanity, of mercy, or of justice. To commit acts of this nature requires a fanaticism and wickedness that is beyond our normal contemplation."

As I have previously noted, one of the most difficult aspects of my job as a risk manager and security consultant is to get good people to understand that evil does exists. No greater evil exists than that in the individual who enters a school, church, office building, or theater and pulls out a weapon and begins shooting innocent people, often not knowing any of their victims. These active shooters are pure evil and show no mercy. It takes a special kind of evil to walk into Sandy Hook Elementary School and murder twenty six and seven-year-old kids. I have stated in this book many times that "survival is a mindset, not a skill set"; the sooner you understand and accept the fact that evil does exist, the better prepared you can be to react and defend yourself against it.

Billions of dollars have been invested to provide law enforcement officers with additional force, training, and weaponry to enable them to respond better to this growing threat of active shooters. However, little has been done to address the training needs of the average person who is at the forefront of these events. This is a significant oversight given the statistics that, on average, it takes twelve to fourteen minutes for law enforcement officers to respond, while the average active shooter event is typically over in eight minutes. That is fourteen minutes where the undertrained, and often unprepared, are left to fend for themselves. The vast majority of innocent bystanders will not know what to do to minimize the risks during these critical "minutes that matter."

The training and consulting services I have developed are designed specifically to address this gap, and are rooted in my overwhelming desire to save lives. I strive to modify a person's behavioral response in the face of a threat, while emphasizing that one need not live in fear. Awareness and preparedness provide peace of mind. It's the "not knowing what to do" that causes unnecessary fear.

Hiding Is the Wrong Answer

For years the Department of Homeland Security has marketed the mantra of Run-Hide-Fight in the event you are caught in the middle of an active shooter situation. I have always had a problem with the word "hide." I know their intent is to provide a "one-size-fits-all" answer in responding to an active shooter; however, no two events are the same, and it has been shown in numerous active shooter events that hiding does not work!

The proper response to an active shooter event is: MOVE—do NOT hide!

Hiding under a desk is not a tactical plan that helps anyone...except the shooter. Hiding only makes you an easy target for the killer. Your best course of action in any shooting situation is to move: to RUN. Being able to hit a moving target is a very difficult skill to master. The average hit rate on a moving target is 4 percent! In other words, you have a 96 percent chance of not being shot if you move. Running around the room hoping the shooter runs out of ammunition and then tackling him while he tries to reload is a better option than hiding under your desk.

Kristina Anderson was a survivor of the horrific 2007 Virginia Tech shooting in which thirty-two people were killed and seventeen were wounded. She was shot three times as she attempted to protect herself by hiding under her desk. The desk type was your typical flip-top school desk and plastic chair. Kristina travels the country telling her story of survival. She explains how her desk was the fourth desk in the row located nearest the door. The shooter entered and exited her classroom three times, before finally ending his life in the front of the room. Kristina is an ardent supporter of the message, "Hiding does not work." Could she have escaped by running out the classroom door? We'll never know. However, I am sure that had she known then what she knows now, she would not have kneeled down under her desk, head down, waiting for her turn to be shot.

One of the first news reports on the 2018 Annapolis active shooting event that occurred at the offices of The Capital, a newspaper serving the area, was from Phil Davis, a gazette reporter who was in the office during the event. His account of what he felt is heart-wrenching (with my emphasis added):

> There is nothing more terrifying than hearing multiple people get shot while you're *under your desk* and then hear the gunman reload. I'm a police reporter. I write about this stuff—not necessarily to this extent, but shootings and death—all the time. But as much as I'm going to try to articulate how traumatizing it is to be *hiding* under your desk, you don't know until you're there and you feel *helpless*.

I hate that this reporter felt "helpless" and that he did what most others would do in the same situation, and what most of us have been told to do and what our instinct tell us to do—hide.

If you are unable to escape the area, then and only then should you enter a room, lock the door, and prepare to fight. Preparing to fight means looking for improvised weapons such as scissors, fire extinguishers, pens, large cans, and other blunt instruments that can cause serious bodily injury to the shooter if he tries to enter the room. This is a "proactive" response to a critical incident, not a "passive'" response such as hiding under a desk.

There is no one-size-fits-all approach or response to surviving an active shooter event. No two situations are the same. However, the one thing you can do is to develop a Survival Mindset, which is your greatest weapon. The will to survive is much more important than the skill to survive.

The majority of Americans can do incredible things, and will, if empowered to do so. Just ask Mr. James Shaw Jr. of Nashville, Tennessee, who disarmed an active shooter in a Waffle House in April of 2018. Mr. Shaw was a customer at the South Nashville restaurant when a man walked in and killed four people and injured many others. Shaw said he ran toward the bathroom when the gunfire started. Then, realizing he was trapped, he rushed the shooter, who was reloading, grabbed the hot barrel of the rifle, then disarmed the shooter and threw the gun over the counter. He is credited, and rightly so, with saving numerous lives.

Our law enforcement officers, who are trained in firearms proficiency, have a national hit rate of only 18 percent in police shooting incidents. In other words, police officers miss their target 82 percent of the time! I am confident when I say that most active shooters do not have the training, nor the skill set, of these fine officers. Therefore, your best chance of surviving

an active shooter event is to move. Use the 96 percent probability of NOT getting shot if you move, versus the 100 percent
probability of being shot if the shooter finds you hiding under
your desk.

In the Annapolis incident at The Capital newspaper offices,
the police responded in an unbelievable sixty seconds and ran
directly to the gunfire! The survivors of this tragedy owe a great
deal of gratitude to those brave police officers. They did exactly
what they were trained to do—run to the gunfight and stop the
killing. However, this was an exception! As I have previously
mentioned, the police response time averages twelve to fourteen
minutes, while the average active shooter event lasts less than
nine minutes. Do that math! Surviving an active shooter event
is your responsibility.

Prior to killing five employees and injuring two others
with a shotgun, the Annapolis gunman sent enraged letters
and messages to the newspaper's offices. He was angry at
the paper for publishing an article in 2011 about the shooter
being put on probation for harassing a high school acquain-
tance. What did the office do with the threatening letters?
Were the employees made aware of the threats and the person
responsible? Was the gunman's name and photograph provided to the newspaper staff and employees? With the abun-
dance of "pre-incident indicators," could this attack have been
prevented? I do not have the answers, but if these threatening
letters were sent to your firm, what would be your plan of
action?

In all my years of training counter terrorism teams, SWAT
teams, police and civilians, I have learned that it's awareness,
preparation, and training that provides peace of mind. It's the
"not knowing what to do" that causes unnecessary fear and
panic. With mass shootings becoming more frequent and more
deadly, people should be thinking about what to do if they're

caught in an active shooter event. Knowledge creates confidence, and confidence produces action. Action keeps you alive!

The Phobic Response to Extreme Violence

In his book *On Killing: The Psychological Cost of Learning to Kill in War and Society*, author David Grossman details the physiological processes involved with killing another human being. In it, he reveals that most people have a phobic-level response to violence, and that soldiers need to be specifically trained to kill. In addition, he details the physical effects that violent stresses produce on humans, ranging from tunnel vision, auditory exclusion, perception of time, changes in sonic perception, reduced motor skills, loss of bladder or bowel control, and post-traumatic stress disorder.

The only way to avoid the natural reaction to extreme violence, which is to freeze in fear or disbelief, is to be trained to react. Active Shooter Response Training is critical to instill the knowledge and confidence needed to react under extreme duress. Businesses, hospitals, schools, and warehouses all need to have active shooter response training. When done correctly, people will no longer huddle in fear, but take active measures to survive.

As a Security Consultant and Risk Manager, my goal is to empower others to be active participants in their own survival. By providing them with the knowledge and the awareness to react when violence strikes, they learn to become more self-reliant; they become their own hero, because they know the police may *not* arrive in time. In an emergency, everyone is going to be trying to save themselves; you better know what to do!

A Plan of Action based on fundamentals may still fail without clear communication before, during, and after a critical incident. What is said and how it's said plays an important role in the action plan. Be sure the language used to communicate is clear and concise. The plan should include the **avoid, deny, defend** (A.D.D moniker), which is taught by the Advanced

Law Enforcement Rapid Response Training (ALERRT) Center at Texas State University.

The ALERRT Center is internationally recognized as employing the foremost experts in collecting data and providing information on active shooter incidents. The ALERRT Center is funded by the Department of Justice, and their training courses are free to police departments across the country. The ALERRT curriculum focuses on teaching police officers and first responders how to react and stop an active shooter event. The center has trained thousands of police officers on how to run to the gunfire. ALERRT teaches, "You have to first stop the killing; then stop the dying."

In their Civilian Response to the Active Shooter Event course, the ALERRT center teaches participants to go through the following progression to stay alive: AVOID, DENY, DEFEND.

- AVOID the shooter at all costs. If you know the shooter's location, create as much distance from the shooter as possible. Get off the X! Leave! Run! Get Out!
- DENY the shooter access to your location if you are unable to create distance. Lock the door; secure it with belts, neckties, tables or chairs—anything to prevent the shooter from gaining access.
- DEFEND yourself should the shooter gain access to your space. Use any improvised weapon you can find and if need be, defeat the shooter using your hands and your survival mindset. If you are with others, devise a plan to attack the shooter should he enter your space. Swarm the shooter. Attack the gunman's vulnerable areas, such as his eyes, throat, knees, and groin.

Communication during a critical incident is critical and should include all employees, customers and visitors. Use plain

English to notify everyone in the building of the threat, thereby allowing them to take decisive action.

Every active threat situation will unfold differently. No two active shooter events are the same. By being proactive and implementing sound training strategies, businesses can be prepared and respond immediately to an active shooter. Companies can lessen the risk from an active shooter event by teaching employees that the first response should be to move (RUN) away from the threat.

Data shows that almost half of all active shooter events end before the police arrive on the scene. You have to own that time! Aggressive actions by the potential victims have been shown to reduce the number of casualties that occur during an attack. If you are well prepared to react, you are more likely to survive and save the lives of others.

Be the Sheepdog! Train hard! Commit to maintaining and enhancing your "situational awareness." Develop that "survival mindset." Remember to move in the event of an active shooter. Travel safety is your responsibility. Know the ground truth; stay vigilant; have a plan; and above all else, STAY SAFE.

Appendix 1
STAY SAFE GUIDELINES (SSG)

CHAPTER 1: SURVIVAL MINDSET

SSG: "Survival is not a skill set; it's a mindset." To survive a violent encounter or a high-risk, high-threat situation your mental attitude is more important than the weapon you have on hand.

SSG: Get Off the X—Action is survival; inaction is death. The best thing you can do if you're caught in a violent encounter is, Move! Walk away! Run! Get off the X! If you find yourself in the middle of an active shooter event or a violent encounter, running is your best chance to survive.

SSG: Trust your gut instinct. You are not paranoid. Do not ignore that inner voice that is warning you, something is not right!

SSG: If a predator has a gun and you're not under his control, always RUN! The chance of him hitting a running target (you) is 4 in 100 shots (4 percent); even then, it probably won't be a fatal wound. Run, preferably in a zigzag pattern, away from the threat. You have a 96 percent chance of not being shot!

SSG: "Violence is almost never the answer, but when it is, it's the only answer!" (Tim Larkin).

SSG: Random violence happens! We do not have to embrace it, condone it, like it, or even understand it; but we must accept that it is a part of our lives. People hurt other people, sometimes fatally. Evil exists.

SSG: Those who survive violent encounters do so because they have the mindset and the intent to do real harm to another human-being when real harm is what's required.

CHAPTER 2: SITUATIONAL AWARENESS
SSG: Having good Situational Awareness is the best thing to avoid any crisis or violent encounter.

SSG: The way you carry yourself can determine if you will be singled out or ruled out as a target for violent criminals! Walk with a purpose—head high, shoulders back, aware of your surroundings.

SSG: Have a "Code Word" that tells your children danger is near and for them to evacuate the area and call 911. Have another "Code Word" that indicates you are under duress. If you use this duress word in a phone conversation, the receiver will know you need immediate help.

CHAPTER 3: YOUR EDC (EVERYDAY CARRY)
SSG: The three must-have items on you at all times: a flashlight, multi-tool, and a tactical pen.

SSG: Have a Go-Bag in your home in case of emergency. Pack it with water, food (freeze-dried camp meals or military-style MREs), fixed-blade knife, flashlight, fire starter, Chem-Lights, lighter, 550 cord, hand axe, medical kit (to include a good tourniquet and blood clotter), pen/paper, change of clothes, and cash.

SSG: "It is better to have it and not need it than need it and not have it!" This philosophy can be the difference between staying safe or being a victim.

SSG: If a robber asks for your wallet or purse—do NOT just hand it to them. Throw it towards them, but far enough away that he has to move. Chances are he is more interested in your money, than in you. When he goes to pick it up—RUN. It's very difficult to hit a moving target with a handgun.

SSG: Always keep a tactical flashlight with you and use it at night. Having a light allows you to see better in the darkness, but it can also be a deterrent to would-be criminals. Because law enforcement officers are usually the only ones shining flashlights down alleys and under cars, if you're shining your light as you walk to your destination or back to your car, the bad guys will probably think you're a cop. If worst comes to worst and you do get jumped, you can use the tactical flashlight as a defensive tool by shining the powerful beam of light into his eyes, momentarily blinding him, or even by hitting him with the beveled edge.

SSG: If you choose to be a Sheepdog and want to get a Concealed Handgun License (State laws vary greatly), know that with this privilege comes great responsibility. You must train continuously. If you're not regularly training to shoot quickly and accurately, at a minimum of five hundred rounds per quarter (2,000 rounds-a-year), you are not training enough; you will be more of a danger to yourself and to others by carrying your weapon.

CHAPTER 4: TRAVEL SECURITY

SSG: You are never without your cellphone. Therefore, use it as an integral part of your security plan by downloading apps that can save your life.

SSG: Get good intelligence! Know the Ground Truth on the country you are visiting. Know the customs, cultures, predicted weather for your visit, celebrations and national holidays. The US State Department has multiple links which provide detailed information on every country you may wish to visit.

SSG: Have a communication plan in place with family and friends before you leave. If you fail to check in at the designated times, they will know you need assistance.

SSG: Nothing you leave in the hotel room is safe, not your laptop, data on any electronic device, USB drives, or your credit cards. Ask the concierge desk to lock up your valuables while you're out.

SSG: When booking a hotel room, request a room between the third and sixth floor—away from the stairwell. Most fire trucks have ladders to reach up to the sixth floor.

SSG: Most fatalities in an airplane crash don't happen from the impact, but rather from smoke inhalation. When possible, reserve a seat within five rows of an emergency exit.

SSG: The most dangerous aspect of traveling is the taxi ride. Once you enter a taxi, you're placing yourself in a very vulnerable position—you are in a stranger's car with your safety in the driver's hands. Be sure to know which taxi cabs are legitimate and never take a cab from someone who solicits you—you call for the cab. If possible, prior to travel, arrange pickup with a reputable transportation company and have them provide a photo ID of the driver and the vehicle.

CHAPTER 5: HOME & VEHICLE SECURITY

SSG: Think like a criminal! Walk around your home and your neighborhood during the day and at night with the mindset of robber deciding on which house he would choose to rob. Use that information to make sure your home isn't the one he would choose.

SSG: Doorbell cameras. This is an inexpensive and very effective deterrent; criminals do not want to be seen and recorded on camera. These systems send reliable alerts to your smartphone when visitors arrive or when packages are delivered. It allows you to talk to visitors through its speakers, and can record suspicious activity, day or night, around your entryway.

SSG: Picking a lock is an easy skill to master! Be sure your exterior doors have good, solid, and sturdy locks.

SSG: Develop and rehearse your family Home Defense Plan.

SSG: Set up a Safe Room in your home. This room should have an inexpensive flip phone with 911 pre-set with a push of the 1 button, a spare car fob to engage your car alarm to create noise and confusion for the home invader, weapons or improvised weapons, small medical bag with prescriptions and trauma dressings, a flashlight, and an emergency ladder if room has a window.

SSG: Women have a tendency to get into their cars after shopping, dining out, or a day at work and sit for a while re-doing their makeup, checking their phones, compiling lists or going through their purses—with their car doors unlocked. Don't do this! A predator may be watching you, and this is the perfect opportunity for him to jump into your passenger seat, put a gun to your head and demand you drive away with him.

SSG: If someone does get into your car and puts a gun to your head, DO NOT DRIVE OFF! Instead, push on the gas pedal and crash into anything, wrecking the car and causing the air bags to deploy. As soon as the car crashes, bail out and run. This is a much better option than having them find your lifeless body in a remote location.

SSG: If you are ever thrown into the trunk of a car, kick out the back tail lights and stick your arm out the hole and start waving like crazy. The driver won't see you, but everybody else will.

SSG: In the event that you are kidnapped or held prisoner, it is important to remember your greatest chance to escape is in the first hour; consequently, your greatest chance of being injured by your kidnapper is also in the first hour.

SSG: Restraints such as handcuffs, duct tape, rope, and flex-ties can be overcome. Learn how and practice often.

CHAPTER 6 : COMMUNITY SECURITY (CHURCHES & SCHOOLS)

SSG: Training makes a difference. Conduct Active Shooter Response Training for your entire office, church, or school staff. Fear comes from not knowing what to do in a critical situation.

SSG: Remember, hiding does not work! It only makes you an easy target.

SSG: There is no "one-size-fits-all" security plan. Every school, church, office, warehouse is different and requires its own security plan. Hire a professional security consultant to help in developing a plan for you; then, communicate the plan to your people.

SSG: Every member of a security team needs to do an honest self-assessment and understand where their weaknesses are and what their true skill sets are.

SSG: Five items you should keep in your desk, especially schoolteachers: hammer, box cutter, screwdriver, tactical pen, and a fire extinguisher. All of these items will not raise suspicion and are easily explained away.

SSG: A vast majority of security matters can be resolved with a smile and a handshake. Don't be too quick to go "hands on," always attempt to de-escalate the situation; don't make matters worse by being overly aggressive.

CHAPTER 7: CORPORATE SECURITY

SSG: Create a Culture of Safety with weekly security tips or security notices; invent games that develop security awareness in your employees.

SSG: Senior management must develop a portal in which employees can report suspicious activity or intelligence/information on possible threats.

SSG: Businesses MUST have a written Active Shooter Response Plan, that plan needs to be communicated to its employees, and training programs must be implemented.

SSG: Hire a seasoned professional with experience in counterterrorism, physical security, and cybersecurity as your CSO; these usually come from government agencies such as the FBI, CIA, or USSS.

SSG: A good Executive Protection program will increase the productivity of the Principal by allowing him to stay focused on his work no matter where that work takes him. This productivity supports the return on investment (ROI) on the security program and it keeps the board members happy knowing their CEO is safe and out of harm's way.

SSG: Teaching "tradecraft" skills to senior executives will be fun, yet arm them with skills that could potentially save their lives.

SSG: The difference between a bodyguard and a Personal Protection Officer (PPO) is a bodyguard specializes in muscles and has a gun; a PPO is better prepared to identify vulnerabilities and threats before it materializes. He also has a gun, but he knows his brain is his most important and lethal weapon.

SSG: Crisis Action Plans, Continuity of Operations Plan, and Contingency Plans are essential for any company that wants to survive in today's more dangerous world.

SSG: If you ever encounter an IMPROVISED EXPLOSIVE DEVICE, which includes pipe bombs, hand grenades, suicide vests, or even Molotov cocktails, you'll need to create distance and angles from the device.

SSG: You don't let strangers into your home, so don't let strangers into your business. Don't assume outside contractors have been vetted or have had a background check. Check their credentials and their identification closely before you allow them access.

CHAPTER 8: SPECIAL EVENT SECURITY

SSG: A Layered Security Approach is the best defense when securing your special event, whether large or small, public or private.

SSG: Plan for worst-case scenarios—extraordinary crimes, violence by protestors, a possible terrorist attack, and natural disasters—but also be thoroughly prepared to deal with ordinary crimes and incidents, such as a lost child, fights, an unattended bag, drunkenness, or small protests.

SSG: Bring your Security Consultant, who is experienced in Special Event Security Planning, in early for the event planning process. Today's security is complex because the threats are complex.

SSG: Hire a seasoned professional with experience in counterterrorism, physical security, and special event security planning. This professional should also possess outstanding interpersonal and liaison skills ,which are necessary for planning small or large special events, as they involve multiple agencies and jurisdictions.

MINUTES MATTER

SSG: AVOID – DENY – DEFEND – Actions to take if you find yourself in an active shooter event. AVOID the shooter. Move! If you cannot escape the area, find a room and DENY the shooter access by moving furniture, using telephone cords, belts, or neckties to tie the door shut. After you have denied access, look for items that can be used as improvised weapons to DEFEND yourself and others should the shooter gain access.

SSG: If a predator has a gun and you're not under his control, always RUN! The chance of him hitting a running target (you) is 4 in 100 shots; even then, it probably won't be a fatal wound. Run, preferably in a zigzag pattern.

SSG: Predators are smart! The "crying baby lure" goes something like this: The attacker plays a recording of a baby crying and puts it on your front porch, or under your bedroom window. When you go out to check on the sound, you become a victim of the assailant.

ACKNOWLEDGEMENTS

Special thanks goes out to all the men and women who self-ishly put on a uniform, military and law enforcement, and put their lives on the line each day as they keep watch over us and protects us from the evils of this world. And to the moms and dads who raised their children to be selfless, honorable, and swear an oath to protect and serve.

Thank you to all the FBI special agents in the field conducting investigations, interviews, surveillances, managing informants, and arresting those who wish to do us harm. You are living the *Fidelity, Bravery, and Integrity* code of the greatest law enforcement agency in the world—the FBI.

Thanks to the men of the FBI's Hostage Rescue Team—no greater group of warriors exists on the face of the planet. Your selfless dedication, courage under fire, quiet professionalism, and bravery exhibited in the Global War on Terror are qualities few will ever know. I am humbled and honored to have been your teammate. Servare Vitas!

Thank you to Tony Jeary (the Results Guy) and his staff for helping me make this project a reality, along with Ben, John, and Ayesha.

To Larry Carpenter and his staff at Carpenter's Son Publishing for their outstanding work in making this into something you can hold.

To Betsy Wilder, the finest editor I never had to pay, and the best mother-in-law a man could wish for. Thank you for all your advice, counsel, and edits to make this book so very much better.

To the men and women who train daily to maintain their skill set and to keep their edge sharp to help defend those in need when the "Wolves" come to visit the "Sheep." Knowing you and the thousands of others like you are among us, to defend the helpless, allows me to sleep soundly in my bed. Warriors like Chris "Dutch" Moyer, Brian Harpole, Chris Grollnek, Steve Moses, Allan McBee, Justin Davis, Brad Tuttle, Chris Mills, Dan Flood, Charlie Sanchez, Jeff Muller, Brig Barker, Danny Coulson, Kevin Kolbye, Dave Shellenberger, Derek Bailey, Matt Morgan, Whit Darnell, Scott Ward, Jim Smith, Mario Verna, Tim Denny, Tony Smith, and too many others to name—but you know who you are. These men and those like them are always "at the ready" to bring violence upon those who wish to do us harm.

To the amazing (and quite large) Shaffer Family—the love and special bond we all share is a rare and unique gift. I thank God each day for the love from this amazing family and the support you have shown throughout my entire life. I love each and every one of you!

Finally to my wife, Dotty—the most beautiful and amazing woman I know. She suffered through my years on HRT with midnight "callouts" taking me to places where she knew I'd be in harm's way. Her courage, commitment, and loyalty are unmatched. This book would not be possible without her encouragement, support, and unwavering love. My wife and the millions of other spouses who have cried themselves to sleep never knowing if and when their loved ones would return—they are the true "Warriors" and the bravest of all.

God bless our peacekeepers! Stay Safe.

ABOUT THE AUTHOR

G reg Shaffer served in the Federal Bureau of Investigation (FBI) for twenty years, including six years on their elite Hostage Rescue Team or HRT.

Mr. Shaffer supervised, developed, and implemented the security plan for the 2011 NFL Super Bowl hosted in Dallas, Texas, while assigned as a supervisor on the FBI's North Texas Joint Terrorism Task Force. His FBI career also included assignments in the San Francisco Field Office, where he was a member of their SWAT team and assigned to a multi-agency drug task force. He also served at the National Counter Terrorism Center (NCTC) in McLean, Virginia, and was selected by the Director of the FBI to be the first FBI Legal Attaché assigned to the US Embassy in Budapest, Hungary.

Mr. Shaffer started his professional career as a line-officer in the United States Coast Guard where he served for eleven years and commanded the Coast Guard Cutter Point Steele. He also served as the Commandant's Liaison Officer to the US House of Representatives, and a Deck Watch Officer aboard the US Coast Guard Cutter CHASE (WHEC 718).

He holds a bachelor of science degree in management from the United States Coast Guard Academy, as well as a master's certificate from the Australian Institute of Police Management, and he is a graduate of the FBI Academy in Quantico, Virginia.

Mr. Shaffer currently is the founding partner in SHAF-FER SECURITY GROUP (www.shaffersecuritygroup.com), a global security and tactical training specialty firm based in Dallas, Texas.

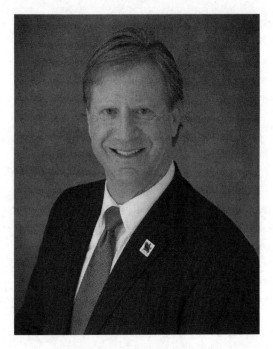

Author: Greg Shaffer; Photo Credit: Jake Felts Photography

SHAFFER SECURITY GROUP (SSG)

The Shaffer Security Group leads the way in Security Consulting and Risk Assessment services for organizations throughout the United States and abroad. Our team of experts protects our clients from potential threats that could harm their business, enterprises, interests, and staff members.

From special event security planning, where we create strategic security plans that have ensured the safety of over 100,000 civilians and staff members, to situational awareness training for personnel to proactively think about security threats and risks and how to properly respond to an active threat, our goal is to help our clients create a unique strategic security plan and solution that will span their entire operation.

There is no suitable word for what we do. Traditional security does not fit; our team is composed of FBI Hostage Rescue Team Operators, Law Enforcement Officers, Intelligence Officers, and Special Military Operations Officers. Security response services does not seem proactive enough. Our job is to prevent incidents from happening; responding to a threat after the fact means there was a weakness in the security planning. We see ourselves as security planners, certainly not as a security guard company.

Our services include: Risk Management, Security Consulting, Special Event Security Planning, Active Shooter Response Training, Executive Protection and Executive Protection Training, Tactical Firearms Training, Travel Safety Courses, and International and Domestic Investigations.

Visit us on our Website @ www.shaffersecuritygroup.com
FaceBook@Shaffer.Sec.Group
Instagram@ShafferSecurityGroup
Twitter @ShafferGroup

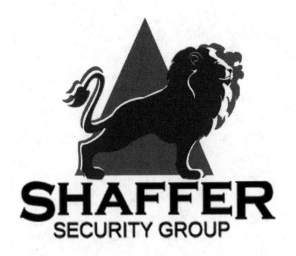

REFERENCES

American Institute on Domestic Violence. 2001. "Domestic Violence in the Workplace Statistics." www.aidv-usa.com/statistics.htm (accessed July 1, 2006).

Book, Angela, Kimberly Costello, and Joseph A. Camilleri. 2013. "Psychopathy and Victim Selection: The Use of Gait as a Cue to Vulnerability." *Journal of Interpersonal Violence.*

Bureau of Labor Statistics, US Department of Labor. "National Census of Fatal Occupational Injuries in 2016." USDL-17-1667 (December 19, 2017).

Cooper, J. 1989. *Principles of Personal Defense.* Boulder: Paladin Press.

De Becker, Gavin. *The Gift of Fear.* New York: Little, Brown, 1997.

Elder, Larry. 2018. "How Many Lives Are Saved By Guns—And Why Don't Gun Controllers Care?" Investors Business Daily (March).

FBI Uniform Crime Reporting Statistics. 2015. Crime in the United States, Property Crime, Criminal Justice Information Services.

Fuschillo, Alanna. 2018. "The Troubling Student-to-Counselor Ratio That Doesn't Add Up." Committee for Economic Development (May).

Grossman, David. 2004. On Combat: The Psychology and Physiology of Deadly Conflict in War and in Peace. New York: PPCT Research Publications.

Larkin, Tim. 2017. *When Violence is the Answer—Learning How to Do What It Takes When Your Life Is at Stake.* Little, Brown and Company, New York.

Musu-Gillette, L., A. Zhang, K. Wang, J. Zhang, J. Kemp, M. Diliberti, and B.A. Oudekerk (2018). Indicators of School Crime and Safety: 2017. National Center for Education Statistics, US Department of Education, and Bureau of Justice Statistics, Office of Justice Programs, US Department of Justice. Washington, DC.

Pham, Tammy B., Lana E. Schapiro, John Majnu, and Andrew Adesman. 2015. "Weapon Carrying among Victims of Bullying." *Pediatrics* 140, no. 6 (December).

Silver, James, Andre B. Simons, and Sarah Craun. "Study of Pre-Attack Behaviors of Active Shooters in the United States Between 2000 and 2013." US Department of Justice, Federal Bureau of Investigation (June 2016).

Statista: The Statistics Portal. 2017. "Percentage of Households in the United States Owning One or More Firearms from 1972 to 2018" (October) https://www.statista.com/statistics/249740/percentage-of-households-in-the-united-states-owning-a-firearm/.

Swanberg, J., and T. K. Logan (2005). "Domestic Violence and Employment: A Qualitative Study." *Journal of Occupational Health Psychology* 10, no. 1: 3–17.

US Department of Justice, Federal Bureau of Investigation. "A Study of Active Shooter Incidents in the United States between 2000 and 2013" (September 2013).

Van Horne, Patrick, and Jason A. Riley. 2014. *Left of Bang*. Black Irish Entertainment.